Essentials of Accident and Emergency Care

John Lourie
BM PhD FRCS

Consultant Orthopaedic and ...
Milton Keynes Hospital

Anthony Bradlow
MD MRCP DCH

Consultant Rheumatologist
Battle Hospital, Reading

Mary Sutters
RGN RCNT DipN

Senior Nurse, Accident and Emergency Department
Royal Berkshire Hospital, Reading

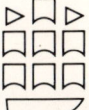

CHURCHILL LIVINGSTONE
EDINBURGH LONDON MELBOURNE AND NEW YORK 1987

CHURCHILL LIVINGSTONE
Medical Division of Longman Group UK Limited

Distributed in the United States of America by
Churchill Livingstone Inc., 1560 Broadway, New York,
N.Y. 10036, and by associated companies,
branches and representatives throughout the world.

First published/1987

ISBN 0 443 03903 8

British Library Cataloguing in Publication Data
Lourie, John
  Essentials of accident and emergency care.
  1. Emergency nursing
  I. Title   II. Bradlow, Anthony
  III. Sutters, Mary
  610.73′61   RT120.E4

Library of Congress Cataloging in Publication Data
Lourie, John.
  Essentials of accident and emergency care.
  Bibliography: p.
  Includes index.
  1. Emergency nursing. I. Bradlow, Anthony.
II. Sutters, Mary. III. Title. [DNLM: 1. Emergencies—
nurses' instruction. 2. Emergency Service, Hospital—
nurses' instruction. 3. Traumatology—nurses'
instruction. WX 215 L892e]
RT120.E4L68 1988   616′.025   87-9380

Produced by Longman Singapore Publishers (Pte) Ltd.
Printed in Singapore

Essentials of Accident and Emergency Care

Preface

When the learner nurse is first allocated to a busy Accident and Emergency (A & E) Department she is understandably anxious. So much seems to be going on, and everyone but she has a job to do and knows what he is doing. She can feel left out, incompetent and positively in the way.

This book has been written to give the learner nurse confidence by explaining *what* is going on, and *why*. This will enable her to care for and communicate effectively with her patients, so gaining the cooperation necessary for them to participate in their care.

Patients come to A & E because they are *ill* or *injured*, so the book is divided into these two sections. Within each, common types of illness or injury are dealt with in individual chapters, cross-referenced where appropriate. You may find the practice in your hospital differs from the regimes of patient care described in this book. Often there is no one 'best way' of doing things, but the learner must understand why things are done the way they are.

The nurse is the one person who is with the patient throughout his time in A & E. The receptionist, doctor, porter and radiographer may all be in contact with him at different times but it is the nurse who must ensure that all the patient's needs have been considered. For every patient a nursing assessment should be made and recorded. A formal documentation system may be used, or a simple check-list. If no such system operates in your Department this is still a useful way to approach your patient's care.

Although the nurse does not make a diagnosis, her understanding of significant signs and symptoms is essential. Her knowledge will enable her to provide suitable care and pass on relevant information. In so doing she helps to ensure that the patient gets the most accurate diagnosis and suitable treatment.

In the text the female or the male gender is often used alone: it is too cumbersome to say 'him or her' throughout, but the book refers equally to *all* nurses and *all* patients.

Milton Keynes and Reading, 1987

J.L.
A.B.
M.S.

Acknowledgements

This book could not have been written without the help of those who have taught us in the past, the experience of caring for ill and injured patients, the tolerance of our families and the patience of our publishers. We gratefully acknowledge our debt to them all.

Contents

PART 2. Injured Patients

PART 1

Ill patients

1 The ill patient in the Accident and Emergency Department

The patient attending the Accident and Emergency Department (A & E) may be:
— unconscious or drowsy
— confused or violent
— in pain
— unable to move one or more limbs
— having difficulty in breathing.
This may be due to:
— drug overdose or poisoning
— heart attack
— stroke
— epileptic attack
— complication of diabetes
— asthma
— unrecognised injury.
Patients may have been brought by relatives or by ambulance to the Department, or may have found their way alone. In inner-city areas many people use A & E as a general practice for minor complaints. Some attenders and their relatives and friends are aggressive, abusive or violent, demanding immediate attention. Some are vagrants. They may be unable to give a proper account of themselves or their symptoms. The variety and complexity of these problems pose great challenges to the nurse.

> **Throughout the patient's time in A & E the nurse has a responsibility to care for the patient's physical, psychological and social needs.**

Her role on receiving patients is to:
• **Identify** the general problem for which the patient is attending A & E
• **Assess** his immediate needs
• **Obtain** information from relatives or attendants about the patient's social circumstances, current medications and past/current illnesses

- **Undress** the patient fully and put in a gown preparatory to medical examination, causing the minimum of discomfort and taking account of the need for privacy, modesty and warmth
- **Make** and **record** observations of *pulse, blood pressure respirations, temperature* and *neurological state*
- **Ensure** a vomit bowl and urinal or bedpan are available
- **Save** and routinely **test** any urine, vomit or faeces the patient passes
- **Deal** as far as possible with the questions of the patient and the relatives
- **Talk** *to* the patient, not *over* him, even if he does not respond. Invite relatives to sit with the patient
- **Repeat** the observations of pulse, blood pressure, respiration and temperature if there is a delay before the doctor is available
- **Alert** the nurse in charge immediately if there is any change or sudden deterioration in the patient's condition
- **Consider** pressure areas in susceptible patients (especially the elderly and the paralysed) who may have been lying in one position for some time prior to admission
- **Ensure** examination equipment including neurological and rectal trays is available for the doctor, together with the recordings you have made
- **Remain** with the patient during the examination, and assist the doctor
- **Be prepared** to explain investigations and procedures to the patient
- **Give drugs** only from a *written* order; always follow correct checking procedure
- **Withhold** any food or drink from the patient until the doctor has been consulted.

> **Never leave a patient unattended and out of sight behind screens**

> **If the patient is on a trolley always ensure the cot-sides are in position**

Three possible outcomes of attendance at A & E are:
- *discharge* from hospital (sometimes with instructions to visit the GP or attend an out-patient clinic)
- *admission* to hospital for investigation or treatment, or to a short-stay ward for observation
- *death*, in which case the relatives will need particular care, information and support (see Appendix B).

The nurse has a major role in making arrangements, and in communicating with the patient, relatives and professional colleagues. This ensures that the transfer or discharge of the patient and his belongings is efficiently performed with the appropriate documentation.

2 Cardiopulmonary resuscitation

This term describes the emergency process of re-establishing the oxygen supply to the brain, by restoring breathing and circulation when these have abruptly ceased (cardiopulmonary arrest, Chapter 3).

Resuscitation is a team effort. The outcome can be successful only if every team member is totally familiar with his or her role. A standard procedure followed in all cases allows maximal efficiency. The team usually has five members: 2 doctors, 2 nurses and a porter to help with equipment. Two extra nurses for the first few minutes can be a help; more than this get in the way.

As a learner you will probably assist during a cardiac arrest. Watch what people are doing so you can see the importance of *team-work*. Observe that each person has a specific role.

Cardiopulmonary resuscitation is a practical skill easily lost if not performed regularly. Equipment and personnel must be constantly ready for a resuscitation emergency.
- Know where the equipment is
- Know how it works
- Make sure *daily* it is working
- Practise resuscitation procedures regularly.

Assessment

Recognition of need for resuscitation
- Cardiac arrest can be recognised by:
  - loss of consciousness
  - cessation of breathing
  - stiffening or loss of muscle tone
  - dilated pupils
  - absent "central" pulse (carotid, femoral)
- Respiratory arrest is the same, except the pulse remains.

"Crash Call"
- Often advance warning from ambulance that collapsed patient is being brought in
- In A & E, dial crash call number and say *exactly* where you are phoning from.

Preparations
- lie patient flat; remove false teeth
- give a firm thump on the chest. This:
  - (a) may restore regular heartbeat
  - (b) can dislodge a tracheal or laryngeal foreign body
- move patient to designated resuscitation area in A & E
- note the time precisely
- check equipment ready:
  - endotracheal tubes (various sizes)
  - lubricating jelly
  - laryngoscope
  - prime intravenous (i-v) giving set with 4.2% or 8.4% sodium bicarbonate solution
  - switch on monitor/defibrillator and connect electrodes
  - drugs (see below)
  - syringes (2 ml and 10 ml)
  - No. 1 needles.

The A B C of resuscitation
A — Airway
B — Breathing
C — Circulation

A. Airway
- mouth and pharynx cleared by removal of any visible foreign body by carefully probing with a finger
- vomit cleared with suction apparatus
- extend patient's neck:
  - stand behind patient
  - place two fingers under the chain
  - pull forward
- insert Guedel airway.

B. Breathing
- ventilate with Ambu bag and oxygen
- prepare endotracheal tube
  - laryngoscope ready
  - 10 ml syringe to inflate endotracheal cuff
  - 8-10 mm tubes for adults; 4-8 mm for children
  - ensure appropriate connectors to Ambu bag are ready
  - attach oxygen supply tubing to bag.

C. Circulation

1. *Cardiac message* (unless femoral/carotid pulse can be felt)

Technique of cardiac massage
Place heels of both hands on patient's sternum with both arms held straight in front of you. Lean rhythmically on your outstretched arms. Do *five* chest compressions to *one* squeeze of the ventilation bag.

---

2. *I-v cannula*
- inserted for drug administration.

3. *ECG leads*
- attached to chest or all four limbs
- ECG pattern monitored:
  - ventricular fibrillation
  - asystole
  - other rhythm.

4. Prepare drugs
Always check these with second nurse or doctor.
- *adrenaline* — 1 ml of 1:1000 or 10 ml of 1:10000
- *lignocaine* — 10 ml of 1%
- *atropine* — 3-6 ampoules of 600 μg each
- *calcium chloride* — 10 ml of 10%
- *sodium bicarbonate* — 50 ml of 8.4% (or 200 ml in i-v infusion)
- *5% dextrose* i-v infusion as vehicle for drugs.

5. *Restoration of cardiac output*
(a) Correction of arrhythmias
  - *ventricular fibrillation* by defibrillation
    - large amounts of electrode gel or gel pads required
    - stand well back from patient
    - drugs given: lignocaine
      adrenaline
      bicarbonate
    - defibrillator recharged.
Cardiac massage continued if defibrillation not immediately successful.
  - *asystole*
    - drugs given: atropine
      adrenaline
      bicarbonate
      isoprenaline
    - cardiac pacing.

6. *Observe and record*
 — pulse
 — blood pressure   } continually throughout procedure.
 — pupil size and reaction

Post-resuscitation care

1. *Turn* patient semi-prone to prevent airway obstruction, unless still intubated and/or being ventilated.
2. *Check*
    — pulse
    — blood pressure
    — cardiac rhythm on monitor
    — respirations
    — urine output.
3. *Talk* to the patient: he may be able to understand you even if he cannot respond.
4. *Investigations*
    • blood gases and pH (to assess adequacy of patient's breathing)
    • serum potassium (often reduced to dangerously low levels after resuscitation)
    • chest X-ray (to exclude pneumothorax and pulmonary oedema)
    • ECG (to assess heart rhythm, exclude myocardial infarction).
5. *Treatment*
    • dopamine infusion if blood pressure low
    • lignocaine to stabilise heart rhythm.
6. *Relatives*
    Ensure they are given some privacy in a quiet room. If no-one senior is immediately available to talk to them it may be helpful to:
    — ask how much they know about what has happened
    — check patient's personal details (name, age, GP, previous medical history and drugs, hospital attendances)
    — don't build false hopes; assure them everything possible is being done and more information will be given as soon as possible
    — offer the use of a phone, or make call for them to other relatives
    — offer tea/coffee; allow to smoke if requested.

3 Cardiac emergencies

Most cardiac emergencies are "heart attacks" (myocardial infarction or angina); both are due to ischaemia of heart muscle and are managed similary in A & E. The other major cardiac emergency — cardiac failure — usually presents as an acute respiratory problem.

MYOCARDIAL INFARCTION

Recognition
- chest pain
- difficulty with breathing (dyspnoea)
- occasionally unconsciousness.

Cardiac pain is severe, crushing and felt deep in the centre of the chest. It may be described as "indigestion" by the patient. The pain may pass into the jaws, arms (especially the left) and to between the shoulder blades. Vomiting and sweating frequently occur.

Assessment
- pulse
- blood pressure
- respirations
- colour of face, tongue, fingers
- note any drugs given before patient's arrival at A & E: see GP's letter (additional details may sometimes have been written on the envelope)
- urine output
- level of consciousness.

Emergency investigations
- **ECG**
- **Chest X-ray**
- **Arterial blood gases** (see p.16).

Priority action
- transfer patient to an area or room where resuscitation equipment is available and ready for immediate use

- sit patient upright or in comfortable semi-recumbent position
- give oxygen (24%-40%) by mask
- connect cardiac monitor, positioned facing *away* from patient
- undress patient without allowing him to exert himself
- *reassure patient and relatives by your actions and attitude.*

Watch for complications

Cardiac arrest — indicated by:
- change of body tone (stiffening, flaccidity)
- cessation of breathing
- loss of consciousness
- dilated pupils, absent pulse.

Arrhythmias — indicated by:
- change on ECG monitor
- irregular pulse.

Acute heart failure (see 'Cardiac failure' below) — indicated by:
- dyspnoea
- wheezing
- "bubbly" chest.

Cardiogenic shock — indicated by:
- very low blood pressure
- impaired consciousness
- pallor and sweating.

Drugs often given
Record all drug doses and times (including i-v infusions) while patient is in A & E.

Drug	Action	Route
Morphine Diamorphine	Pain relief	i-v or i-m
Stemetil (prochlorperazine) Fentazine (perphenazine)	Anti-emetic	i-v or i-m
Atropine	Speeds heart	i-v
Beta-blockers	Slow heart Abolish arrythmias	i-v
Lignocaine Disopyramide Verapamil	Abolish arrythmias	i-v

Frusemide	Diuretic: relieves pulmonary oedema	i-v
Narcan (naloxone)	Reversal of respiratory depression caused by opiates	i-v
Dobutamine	Increases cardiac output	i-v infusion

Cardiac pacing may be used for partial or complete heart block.

Transfer/discharge from A & E
Usually to the coronary care unit or to an acute medical ward.

CARDIAC FAILURE

Impaired effectiveness of the heart pump occurs:
— following damage to heart muscle (e.g. myocardial infarction)
— with increased arterial resistance (e.g. hypertension).

Recognition
Fluid accumulates in the lungs and lower extremities leading to:
— dyspnoea (pulmonary oedema)
— lower limb oedema (only if cardiac failure has been present for some time).

Priority action
• Place patient comfortably in semi-recumbent position
• Oxygen by mask (24%)
• Diuretics (e.g. frusemide).

Observations
• pulse
• blood pressure
• respirations
• temperature
• colour of face and tongue.

Investigations
• chest X-ray (to show heart size; pulmonary oedema)
• ECG
• arterial blood gases (see Chapter 4)
• urea and electrolytes.

Transfer/discharge from A & E
Virtually all patients are admitted to the medical ward or coronary care unit.

4 Acute respiratory problems

INTRODUCTION

Respiratory problems may be due to diseases of the heart (see Chapter 3), brain and kidneys, as well as to the more obvious chest conditions.

Recognition
Whatever the cause, patients will show:
— rapid breathing (tachypnoea)
— difficulty with breathing (dyspnoea) or noisy breathing (wheeze, stridor)
— distress, anxiety.
Severely ill patients will also have:
— rapid heart-rate (120-140/minute)
— central cyanosis (blue-tinged tongue)
— confusion, aggression, exhaustion
— coma in most severe cases.

Priority action in the unconscious patient
• Clear airway carefully and turn patient semi-prone
• Ensure the doctor has been called urgently
• **Do not** probe around for a foreign body obstructing the airway: you may convert a partial into a complete obstruction
• Give oxygen by mask
• Transfer patient to a warm, well-lit room with oxygen supply and resuscitation equipment.

Priority action in the conscious patient
• Transfer patient to a warm, well-lit room with oxygen supply and resuscitation equipment
• Sit patient in position he finds most comfortable — often sideways on a trolley with legs handing over the side. **Never leave the patient unattended in this position**
• If required, *carefully* clear the mouth of vomit and foreign bodies (including false teeth)

- Give oxygen by mask but do not force this on the patient. If necessary hold the mask as near to nose and mouth as patient will allow. Ensure tubing is properly connected.
- Check patient's current medications — steroids?
- Emergency drugs commonly used are detailed in the relevant sections below
- Try to reassure the patient and relatives by your actions; answer questions and remain calm
- Leave curtains/door partially open so patient does not feel shut in.

Observations
In all cases record:
- pulse
- blood pressure
- respirations.

Emergency investigations often performed
- Arterial blood gases (P_aO_2 and P_aCO_2) which reflect how adequately the lungs are oxygenating blood and clearing it of carbon dioxide.
  Equipment required:
  Heparinised syringe and needle
  Ice for transporting specimen
  Skin cleansing swab
  Swab (pressure for 5 minutes after sample taken)
- Chest X-ray to exclude pneumothorax (Chapter 4) and pneumonia; may also show aspiration of a foreign body to be the cause of the problem.

```
                      In X-ray:
  •• A nurse must always accompany the patient
  •• Never leave the patient unattended
  •• Be sure you know where the alarm bell and emergency kit are.
```

Alternatively a portable X-ray may be done in A & E.
- Peak flow rate to show severity of wheezing: record best of three attempts.
- ECG to exclude myocardial infarction as cause of the acute respiratory symptoms.

ASTHMA

Asthma is defined as "reversible small airways obstruction".
Expiration is always longer than *inspiration* in asthmatic wheezing.

When receiving/assessing an asthmatic patient:
Ask the relatives (the patient will probably be too breathless):
— what treatment has been given so far? (Particularly, what tablets
   and inhalers have been used?)
— is patient taking steroids?
— has this attack followed a chest infection or possible aspiration
   of a foreign body?
The condition of asthmatic patients can worsen rapidly; **they must
never be left unattended at any time,** particularly in X-ray.

Priority action
• Oxygen by face-mask
• Nebulised salbutamol
• Intravenous aminophylline or salbutamol
• Intravenous hydrocortisone.
Sedative drugs are not given to patients with asthma; agitation or
confusion are *always* due to hypoxia until proved otherwise.
Sedatives lessen the attempt to breathe and can cause sudden
death.

Investigations
• Peak flow rate   } to assess severity
• Arterial blood gases   J of attack
• Chest X-ray (for pneumothorax,   to show severe
   pneumonia and congestive cardiac   associated disease
   failure)   requiring urgent
• ECG (for myocardial infarction)   treatment.

Important points
1. A young child who presents with a first attack of wheezing may
   have inhaled a foreign body.
2. Beware of the patient who shouts "I am dying". Such patients
   are often severely hypoxic; their pleas should not be
   disregarded.

Transfer/discharge from A & E
Ward : Most patients, after initial control of symptoms.
ICU : In severe attack if assisted ventilation required.
Home : In mild attack after observation in A & E and complete
          resolution of symptoms.

Advice to patient on discharge
• Return immediately if wheezing recurs
• Return if symptoms not controlled by normal inhaler dosage
   every four hours
• Avoid any known precipitating factors, e.g. domestic animals.

PNEUMOTHORAX

If air enters the chest between the visceral and parietal pleura (the inner and outer layers of the lining membrane of the chest wall and lungs), the lung collapses. This is a pneumothorax.

Causes
Anything producing a hole in the pleura:
- congenital weakness of the pleura
- rupture of the pleura at a weak point due to abnormally high pressure in the lung (as in asthma)
- penetrating injury (jagged edge of broken rib, stab wound) — in which case air *and blood* are found in the pleural cavity (see Chapter 15)
- erosion of visceral pleura by disease.

Recognition
A patient with a pneumothorax typically:
- is a fit young man (often a smoker) who suddenly experiences a stabbing, poorly localised chest pain and dyspnoea during a football match
- is a known asthmatic who suddenly becomes dyspnoeic without warning, or suffers a sudden worsening of dyspnoea during an asthmatic attack
- has a penetrating chest or abdominal injury (see Chapters 15 and 16) and becomes increasingly dyspnoeic.

The main feature is the **sudden** development of dyspnoea.

Priority action
- Note:
  - distress
  - exhaustion
  - cyanosis
  - respirations
  - pulse
  - blood pressure
- Chest X-ray
- Treatment is by insertion of an underwater seal chest drain:
  - prepare equipment
  - prepare patient
  - explain what is to happen before and at each stage during the procedure, as the patient is often very frightened about both his condition and the proposed treatment.

Procedure (see Figure 1)
- a sterile procedure: the doctor scrubs up and wears gloves, sometimes also gown and mask
- skin preparation

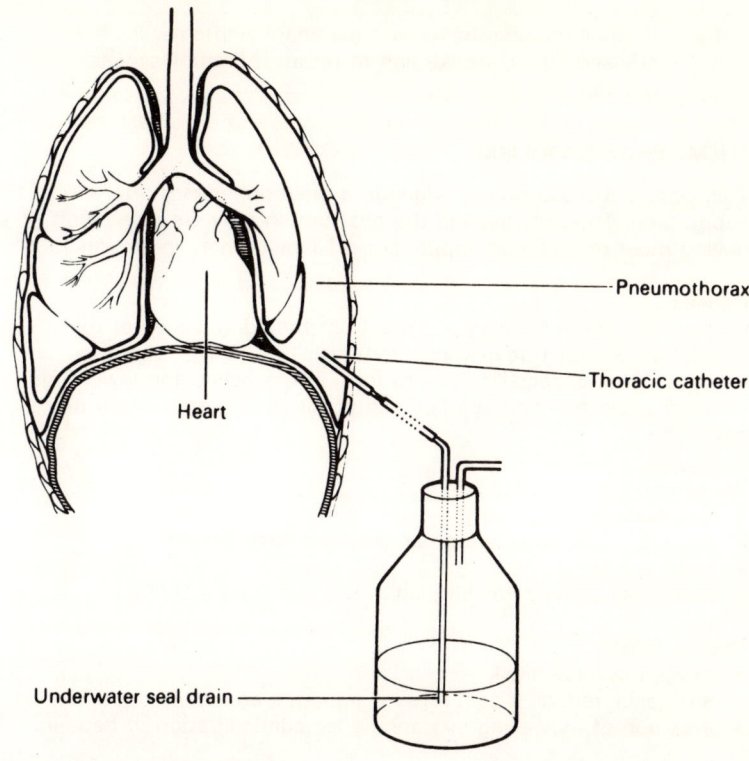

Fig. 1 Underwater seal drain

- local anaesthetic (see Appendix A)
- insertion of drain with introducer (trocar)
- rapidly attach to bottle primed with water standing on floor
- check water is bubbling (ask patient to cough)
- suturing in place of drain
- keyhole dressing and seal with waterproof tape (e.g. Sleek)
- tape tube and fix to bedding
- clamp tube ready for moving
- check chest X-ray for position of tube.

The bottle must at all times be lower than the chest (unless the tube is clamped), or water will siphon back into the chest.

Transfer/discharge from A & E

Ward : Most patients, to await re-expansion of lung and for
physiotherapy.

Home : If small pneumothorax and minimal symptoms. Patient
advised not to smoke and to return if breathlessness
recurs.

PULMONARY EMBOLISM

This occurs if a blood clot lodges in a main pulmonary artery
subdivision. The lung beyond the obstruction may die as a result of
having most of its blood supply cut off ("pulmonary infarction").

Causes
Clots reach the pulmonary arteries from the venous side of the
circulation. A clot ("deep vein thrombosis" or DVT — see also
Chapter 10) is especially likely to form in the pelvic and lower limb
veins of patients who have been immobile in bed after injury or an
operation.

Recognition
- dyspnoea
- pleuritic chest pain (worse on taking a deep breath)
- haemoptysis
- there may or may not be pain in the calf from a DVT.

Priority action
- oxygen by face-mask
- analgesia: reducing pain relieves patient's anxiety
- insertion of indwelling i-v cannula for administration of heparin.

Investigations
- chest X-ray
- blood gases
- ECG.

Transfer from A & E
To medical ward for bed-rest, analgesia and anticoagulant therapy.

PNEUMONIA

"Pneumonia" describes lung infections widespread and severe
enough to impair lung function and threaten life. Patients with
bronchitis (a less severe infection) are rarely so ill or dyspnoeic.

Types of pneumonia

1. *Lobar pneumonia*
- occurs in previously well patients
- reasons for its development unkown
- infection involves whole lobes or segments of lung.

2. *Aspiration pneumonia*
- follows aspiration of infected material (usually vomit) into lungs
- seen in A & E after alcoholic binges, drug overdoses, head injuries. Often only apparent after patient regains consciousness.

3. *Bronchopneumonia*
- occurs in patients debilitated by age or chronic disease (e.g. cancer). Lung infection severe but often patchy.

Recognition
Whatever the type:
- fever
- malaise
- tachycardia
- rapid breathing and dyspnoea.

Examination of chest with stethoscope reveals characteristic crackling sound ("crepitations"). Patients with lobar pneumonia have localised dullness on chest percussion.

Assessment
- Note:
  - respirations
  - pulse
  - blood pressure
  - temperature
  - colour of lips and tongue
  - state of hydration (the dehydrated patient's mouth is dry and tongue coated; oral toilet required).
- Investigations:
  - chest X-ray: confirms the diagnosis
  - blood gases: show reduction in P_aO_2 and P_aCO_2
  - haemoglobin: anaemia?
  - white cell count: indicator of infection
  - urea and electrolytes: patient may be dehydrated
  - blood/sputum cultures: may reveal causative organism.

Priority action
- Oxygen by face-mask (24% or 28% depending on blood gases)
- Rehydration with i-v/oral fluids
- I-v antibiotics.

Transfer from A & E
All patients are admitted to the ward for continued treatment including physiotherapy.

5 Altered consciousness

INTRODUCTION

Confusion and unconsciousness represent the two ends of the spectrum of altered consciousness.

> **Never underestimate confused or unconscious patients;** their condition can deteriorate quickly, often due to airways obstruction. **Never leave these patients unattended.**

Possible dangers to life
- obstruction of airway
- cessation of respiration
- convulsions
- hypoglycaemia
- hypothermia.

The patient cannot be fully assessed until clothing has been removed. Some urgent actions take absolute priority:
- **Maintenance of airway**
- **Control of convulsions.**

Undressing the patient
- Undressing is carried out *carefully*: unsuspected injuries may be present
- Particular attention to *neck* and to *airway*
- Note state of clothing (blood, vomit, urine, faeces, infestation)
- Clothes may have to be cut off
- Check pockets, bags etc. for tablets, medical cards etc.
- Store patient's belongings in a property bag
- Look for bruising/reddening of skin, pressure sores, needle marks, scars (trauma and surgical), dehydration (Chapter 6) and breath odour (alcohol, ketones, "chemical" smell suggesting drug overdose).

Assessment
- Colour of tongue and peripheries (fingers, nose)
- Rectal temperature; if less than 35°C check with low-reading thermometer to exclude hypothermia (see below)
- Pulse — rapid suggests blood loss, hypoxia; slow suggests raised intracranial pressure
- Blood pressure — high suggests cerebral bleeding, hypoxia; low suggests hypothermia, blood loss, drug overdose
- Respirations — rapid suggests chest infection, acidosis; slow suggests head injury, drug overdose
- Pupil size, equality and reaction to light — unequal pupils suggest brain damage; small unreactive pupils are often due to drugs (morphine, heroin), or brain-stem stroke; large (dilated) pupils suggest respiratory failure or drugs such as amphetamine
- Is patient moving all four limbs?
- Level of consciousness, graded as: conscious/responds to commands/responds to pain/no response
- Fits:
  - localised or generalised?
  - duration?
  - incontinence?
  - tongue biting?
  - injury to head?

Investigations
- Fingerprick blood test with glucose oxidase reagent strips to exclude hypo- and hyperglycaemia
- Blood urea, electrolytes, sugar
- Arterial blood gases if infrequent or shallow respiration
- Blood alcohol, salicylate (aspirin) and paracetamol levels
- Blood/urine samples for poison analysis if specific substance suspected
- Skull X-ray (to exclude fracture).

Priority action
- Airway maintained by turning patient semi-prone; endotracheal intubation equipment and oropharyngeal airway must be immediately available
- Breathing maintained by Ambu bag or respirator if necessary
- I-v cannula inserted for drugs and fluids
- Convulsions stopped by giving i-v diazepam (Valium)
- Low blood sugar corrected with i-v glucose
- Dehydration corrected with i-v fluids
- Take measures to restore normal body temperature:
  - cool if pyrexial
  - warm (space blanket or heated room) if hypothermic
- Record pulse, blood pressure and respirations every 15 minutes.

Ask relatives/attendants about:
— episodes of depression/drug overdose
— recent bereavement, job loss, family breakdown, mental disturbance
— alcohol problems (possibility of unsuspected head injury)
— recent ill health (suggesting infection or renal failure)
— epilepsy or other fits.

The confused patient
• Same risks and causes as the unconscious patient
• The hyperactive confused patient may need to be contained and protected from injury and falling in a warm, well-lit room, possibly on a mattress on the floor
• No other patients or valuable/dangerous objects should be nearby
• No sedation will be given until patient has been medically assessed.

Transfer/discharge from A & E
This depends upon the cause and duration of unconsciousness and is dealt with in the individual sections below.

STROKE

A stroke is a rapidly-developing neurological abnormality due to disturbance of the brain's blood supply.
Brain tissue damage results from:
• *haemorrhage* into brain substance or subarachnoid space from bursting of a weak artery
• cerebral arterial blockage (by thrombosis or embolism) causing *cerebral infarction*
• arterial blockage due to very small emboli which are rapidly dissolved, resulting in a "small stroke" *(transient ischaemic attack)* which recovers in a few hours.

Recognition
Cerebral haemorrhage. Known hypertensive patient complains of headache followed by vomiting and loss of consciousness. Pupils are irregular; hemiplegia develops rapidly.
Cerebral infarction. Middle-aged or elderly patient, heavy smoker with history of arterial disease suddenly loses speech and develops hemiplegia without loss of consciousness. Normal blood pressure. ECG may show changes of myocardial infarction.
Subarachnoid haemorrhage. Younger adult suddenly complains of severe headache and then loses consciousness.
Transient ischaemic attack. Middle-aged heavy smoker with history of angina suddenly loses sight in one eye, or power in an arm. Return to normal within minutes or hours.

These four cases represent typical forms of stroke. In reality the features are often not clear-cut, so it may be impossible to distinguish the type of stroke in A & E.

Other conditions resembling stroke
- causing neck stiffness:
  - meningoencephalitis
  - fracture/dislocation of cervical spine.
- causing unconsciousness or hemiplegia:
  - epilepsy
  - head injury (Chapter 14)
  - hypoglycaemia (Chapter 8)
  - brain abscess, meningoencephalitis
  - bleeding into brain tumour.

Priority action
- Airway maintained by lying patient in semi-prone position
- Do *not* tilt patient head-down: this increases cerebral pressure
- Record:
  - pulse
  - blood pressure
  - respirations
  - level of consciousness
  - pupil size/reaction
  - presence/frequency of fits, spontaneous limb movements
- Position patient to protect paralysed limbs and pressure areas.

Transfer/discharge from A & E
Ward : Patients with evidence of cerebral haemorrhage or infarction or subarachnoid haemorrhage.
Home : Patients with transient ischaemic attacks, for later investigation.

SUDDEN LOSS OF CONSCIOUSNESS

Causes
- Cerebral events (fits, stroke)
- Temporarily inadequate cerebral blood supply (faints, Stokes-Adams attacks (heart block), myocardial infarction, postural hypotension — see below)
- Hypoglycaemia
- Non-organic (hysterical) causes.

Recognition
- Ask relatives/attendants about:
  - previous similar events (fits, faints)
  - heart trouble (palpitations, chest pain)

— diabetes
— medications taken.

• Look for:
  — irregular pulse (suggests cardiac arrythmia)
  — postural hypotension, especially in the elderly (more than 30 mmHg difference between lying and standing systolic blood pressure).

Distinguishing 'fits' from 'faints'
Fits:
— occur at any time in any posture
— patient has often learned to recognise aura of impending fit
— unconsciousness lasts up to 30 minutes; sleep often follows recovery.
Faints:
— occur usually in people who are standing up
— slow pulse during and after faint
— unconsciousness rarely lasts more than 2 or 3 minutes.
In both fits and faints the patient can lie still, or have a grand mal convulsion.

Priority action
• **Airway**
• Blood glucose estimation by glucose oxidase reagent strips is *essential;* leads to immediate treatment of hypoglycaemia with i-v glucose if unconscious, then milk and food
• Record:
  — pulse
  — blood pressure
  — respirations
  — neurological observations (see *Assessment,* above)
• ECG if pulse irregular
• Skull X-ray may reveal unsuspected fracture.

Transfer/discharge from A & E
Considerable individual variation depending on many factors, e.g.:
(a) often admitted: patients
  — who remain confused
  — with abnormal neurological signs
  — with repeated loss of consciousness.
(b) often discharged: patients
  — fully recovered after single episode of unsconsciousness.

If discharged:
• faints are rarely investigated unless recurrent
• GP is contacted

- early out-patient appointment may be required
- diabetics referred to specialist clinic.

Advice to patient on discharge
Do not drive or operate machinery until seen in out-patient clinic.

STATUS EPILEPTICUS

Repeated grand mal convulsions without recovery of consciousness between fits. Untreated, may lead to permanent brain damage and death.

Causes
- Commonly due to abrupt withdrawal of anticonvulsant drugs in known epileptic
- Following head injury
- Meningoencephalitis
- Stroke
- Brain tumour (primary or secondary).

Priority action
- Protect **Airway.**
- I-v cannula for drugs, fluids
- Endotracheal intubation, ventilation and oxygen may be required
- Fingerprick blood sugar to exclude hypoglycaemia
- Drugs given include:
  - diazepam (i-v)
  - chlormethiazole (i-v)
  - paraldehyde (i-m)
- General anaesthesia with muscle paralysis may be required if drugs fail to control convulsions — patient will be admitted to ICU.

Transfer from A & E
Patients no longer convulsing are transferred to the ward.

HYPOTHERMIA

This is defined as body core (i.e. rectal) temperature below 35°C. Any patient with a rectal temperature of 35°C on an ordinary thermometer may be much colder; check temperature with a "low-reading" thermometer.

"At risk" of hypothermia are:
- the elderly living alone
- the immobile
- vagrants who "sleep rough"
- drug addicts.

Conditions precipitating hypothermia in these people
- hypothyroidism and hypopituitarism
- alcohol consumption
- infection
- drugs (phenothiazines, tricyclic antidepressants).

Recognition
- patient looks and feels cold
- muscle stiffness and shivering may not occur with profound hypothermia
- pulse is slow, may be irregular
- blue fingers and toes
- rectal temperature below 27°C is associated with unconsciousness and risk of sudden death due to ventricular fibrillation.

Priority action
- Remove wet and soiled clothing; handle patient very gently
- Patient is re-warmed by 0.5 - 1.0°C per hour in foil and a cellular blanket in a warm environment
- Monitor pulse and blood pressure — fall in BP indicates too rapid re-warming
- Oxygen by facemask (24%)
- ECG — sinus bradycardia, shivering artefacts
- Arterial blood gases — raised P_aCO_2, reduced P_aO_2, acidosis
- Blood sugar — abnormally high or low
- Blood urea — often elevated
- Blood cultures — some patients have septicaemia
- Blood drug levels — alcohol, salicylate (aspirin), paracetamol, barbiturate (may reveal cause of hypothermia)
- I-v fluids (warmed to 37°C); severe dehydration often present
- Oral glucose when patient awake.

Transfer from A & E
Patients invariably admitted to the ward for further medical and social investigations.

6 Abdominal problems

ABDOMINAL PAIN

This is a very common cause for attendance at A & E. It can be due to:
— inflammation of an organ (e.g. appendicitis)
— obstruction of the bowel (e.g. strangulated hernia, cancer of the colon)
— perforation of the bowel (e.g. peptic ulcer)
— bleeding into peritoneal cavity (e.g. ruptured ectopic pregnancy)
— stone in the ureter
— urinary infection
— medical causes sometimes (e.g. diabetes, heart attacks).

Recognition
• Pain: may be generalised (all over) or in one place only
• Vomiting (with or without blood)
• Urinary symptoms (pain, frequency, bleeding)
• Bowel symptoms (diarrhoea, constipation, bleeding).

Assessment
Important features in the patient's *history*:
• how long has the pain been present?
• where is it?
• onset sudden or gradual?
• how severe is it?
• constant or intermittent?
• any urinary symptoms?
• any vomiting, diarrhoea or constipation?
• vaginal bleeding or discharge, or menstrual irregularities?
• any other illnesses?
• any medications?

Note:
— pulse
— blood pressure

31

— temperature
— any abnormal swelling: a painful lump may be a hernia (usually groin or umbilical) or an abscess (red, hot and tender, in soft tissue anywhere)
— by the doctor: rectal/vaginal examination.

Investigations
• Test urine for blood, protein, sugar; look for particles of stone
• Haemoglobin
• White cell count (raised in infections)
• Blood sugar (uncontrolled diabetes can cause abdominal pain)
• MSU (urinary infections can cause abdominal pain)
• Chest X-ray (pneumonia can cause abdominal pain)
• ECG (heart attacks can cause abdominal pain)
• IVP (if urinary stone suspected)
• Urea and electrolytes (may be imbalanced through intestinal obstruction or vomiting)
• Serum amylase (test for pancreatitis)
• Cross-match blood (if blood loss has occurred, or major operation planned)
• Test any vomitus for blood and bile.

Priority action
• If the patient is vomiting, *check the airway*; use suction if necessary
• I-v fluids
• Naso-gastric tube, to empty stomach
• Pain relief (though often *not*, as pain is an important clue to diagnosis — see Appendix A).

Transfer/discharge from A & E
Ward   : For most patients with abdominal pain, to await results of investigations, and for later reassessment. Patient must remain "nil by mouth".
Theatre : If diagnosis clear and/or urgent surgery required (e.g. abscess, acute appendicitis, ruptured aortic aneurysm). Routine pre-operative preparation (including consent form) is undertaken in A & E. Ensure patient's possessions are safely bagged, labelled and checked.

HAEMATEMESIS AND MELAENA

Haematemesis is the vomiting of blood, either fresh or altered by digestive juices ("coffee-grounds"). *Melaena* stools contain altered blood. They are tarry black and foul-smelling.
    Heamatemesis and melaena are caused by bleeding from the upper gastro-intestinal tract.

Common causes
- peptic ulceration
- acute gastric erosion (often due to aspirin or prescribed anti-inflammatory tablets)
- gastro-oesophageal varices (varicose veins around the oesophagus where it joins the stomach — these may rupture)
- prolonged vomiting (causes small tears in the stomach)
- clotting disorder (e.g. leukaemia, inherited bleeding diseases).

Patients taking iron tablets have black stools, but testing for blood is negative.

Recognition

Signs of:
- hypovolaemic shock
  - pallor
  - tachycardia
  - hypotension.

History of:
- peptic ulcer
- liver disease associated with varices
- recent high consumption of pain-killers (e.g. for backpain) — can cause gastric erosion
- skin bruising, or bleeding from urethra (suggesting clotting disorder).

Other causes of shock (and their distinguishing features)
- myocardial infarction (abnormal ECG)
- septicaemia (patient is febrile)
- large bowel bleeding (passage of clots per rectum occurs early in the bleed)
- ectopic pregnancy (amenorrhoea and abdominal pain)
- anaphylaxis (recent bee/wasp sting; new medication taken; skin rash).

Priority action
- record pulse, blood pressure and respirations half-hourly
- elevate foot of trolley if hypotensive
- give oxygen by M-C mask
- an i-v infusion is set up
- blood is taken for:
  - grouping and cross-matching
  - full blood count
  - platelets
  - prothrombin time
  - urea and electrolytes
- patient is kept nil by mouth (mouth-wash only should be offered)
- patient should be kept warm

- duty surgical team is notified
- central venous pressure (CVP) line may be inserted in severe bleeding
- monitor urine output
- chest and abdominal X-rays.

Transfer from A & E
To medical or surgical team, depending on arrangements in your hospital.

DIARRHOEA AND VOMITING

These may occur separately or together. The many causes of *diarrhoea* include:

Infection
- viruses
- bacteria (*E. coli*, Shigella, Campylobacter, Salmonella)
- bacterial toxins (e.g. staphylococcal).

Common causes of *vomiting* without diarrhoea include:
- peptic ulceration
- intestinal obstruction
- acute pancreatitis
- bowel ischaemia or infarction in the elderly
- renal or biliary colic
- diabetic ketoacidosis
- infection
- head injury (Chapter 14).

Priority management
- Isolate patients with a possible infective cause of diarrhoea and vomiting
- Use separate room if possible as smell and frequent use of bedpans will be distressing and embarrassing for patient
- Use gloves when handling such patients
- Wash hands after contact with patient
- Do not give oral fluids until patient seen by doctor; offer mouth-wash only
- Note state of hydration
- Record:
  - temperature
  - pulse
  - blood pressure (low in severe dehydration)
  - fluid intake
  - urine output
  - volumes of vomit and faeces

- If patient's skin is soiled, wash and dry carefully. If anal region sore and excoriated, apply bland ointment (e.g. zinc and castor oil)
- Observe your hospital's policy for disposal of infected excretions, soiled linen, etc.

Ask about:
- other people with diarrhoea and vomiting in the family, at the same party, etc.
- foreign travel (unusual infections)
- previous illnesses (especially diabetes)
- drugs currently taken.

Investigations
- stool sample for microscopy and culture; test for blood
- urea and electrolytes (for dehydration/renal function)
- full blood count
- X-ray abdomen (may show pancreatic calcification, intestinal obstruction, bowel perforation).

Treatment
- copious oral fluids if diarrhoea alone
- i-v fluids if vomiting
- naso-gastric tube may be required.

Transfer/discharge from A & E
If admitted, before transfer inform ward of need for barrier nursing/isolation.

Advice to patient on discharge
- Take copious oral fluids
- Take prescribed drugs only until symptoms subside
- Observe strict hygienic precautions (hand-washing, food handling, etc.)
- Contact GP if symptoms persist after 24 hours.

RETENTION OF URINE

This is a common reason for attendance at A & E, usually in older men and due to an enlarged prostate gland. The patient has often had difficulty in passing urine for some months or years.

Recognition
- Inability to micturate
- Lower abdominal pain

Acute retention may occur in cold weather, as a result of constipation, due to drugs (including alcohol), or after operations. The patient may be very distressed and unable to stay still on a stretcher. He may be passing dribbles of urine, so give him a urinal, and allow him to stand up if he wishes.

Assessment
- History, including medications
- General condition (pulse, blood pressure, temperature)
- Enlarged bladder?
- Blood or discharge from urethra?

The doctor will perform a *rectal examination* to feel the size of the prostate gland.

Investigations
- Haemoglobin
- White cell count
- Urea and electrolytes
- Chest X-ray $\Big\}$ as patients are elderly and may need operation
- ECG

Priority action
- Catheterisation (urethral or suprapubic)
- Test urine for blood, sugar, protein
- Send CSU for bacterial culture.

Transfer/discharge from A & E
Usually to ward for further investigations (IVP), to await results of blood tests, trial of micturition, and operation (prostatectomy) if necessary. Being elderly, these patients in particular may be anxious and need reassurance about their home situation. Practical arrangements need to be made with family/friends or by a social worker, for example to cope with an infirm wife or relative left at home, and with pets, and security.

GYNAECOLOGICAL EMERGENCIES

Abdominal pain in women of child-bearing age is often gynaecological in origin, commonly an infection, or a complication of pregnancy, usually impending ("threatened") or actual ("inevitable") abortion.

Recognition
- Bleeding, either vaginally or internally (signs of shock)
- Lower abdominal pain
- Dysuria (burning or stinging on micturition)
- Vaginal discharge
- Painful swelling around vagina
- Rape (see below).

Assessment
- History, including date of last period. Was it normal? Ruptured ectopic (tubal) pregancy is a common cause of severe internal bleeding in a young woman
- Any recent gynaecological surgery (e.g. termination)?
- Pulse, blood pressure, temperature
- Test urine; send specimen of urine and any discharge to bacteriology laboratory
- Examine any blood clots or material passed vaginally, and *save* specimen
- Painful vulval swelling suggests an abscess
- Vaginal examination: cervix dilated in threatened (sometimes) or inevitable (always) abortion. (This may not be done until the patient is seen by the gynaecologist, to keep painful and distressing examinations to a minimum.)

Priority action
- Shock treated if present (i-v fluids; blood grouped and cross-matched)
- Pain relief (see Appendix A)
- Drugs may be given to cause the uterus to contract (ergometrine)
- Antibiotics commenced if infection present or suspected (*after* bacteriology specimen collected)
- *Psychological support and reassurance are essential.* Acute gynaecological or obstetric emergencies are extremely upsetting for the patient. Some patients may be additionally distressed by being examined by a male doctor. Ensure the patient is not exposed more than necessary for examination. This is especially relevant in some ethnic minorities. Remain with the patient throughout the examination.

Transfer/discharge from A & E
Ward   : For most patients with abortions, who are treated with bed-rest and then dilatation and curettage (D & C) when their condition stabilises. Also for infections (e.g. acute salpingitis).

Theatre : For acute blood loss (usually due to a ruptured ectopic pregnancy), or drainage of abscess.

Home   : Occasionally, for strict bed-rest, in the case of a threatened abortion with undilated cervix. GP must be advised of discharge before patient leaves A & E.

Rape
Most patients are seen at a police station. If the woman comes to A & E ensure she is given privacy and supportive female company.
- leave clothing intact

- remain with patient while examined
- do not allow patient to wash until seen by police surgeon
- remain with patient while she is being examined
- offer patient contact number of rape support group: if not known the local Samaritans will be able to help
- if patient's injuries do not warrant admission ensure she has a safe place to go with a supportive friend or relative.

Remember, confidentiality is vital

7 Self-poisoning

Important points
- An epidemic in developed countries — accounts for a significant proportion of all medical emergencies
- Social difficulties often arise in the course of management (see Appendix B)
- Many patients leave notes or telephone friends. A few however (especially the elderly) actively conceal the suicide attempt
- **Self-poisoning must be considered in all unconscious patients, especially those with a previous history of attempted suicide.**

Emergency telephone advice to relatives/friends with patient still at home
- Don't attempt to make patient vomit (he'll probably bite your finger)
- If patient is drowsy or unconscious, dial 999 and ask for an ambulance. Do not bring patient to A & E in the back of a car
- Place patient head-down, with face to one side.

Information needed immediately from patient's friends/relatives/ ambulancemen:
- Has search been made for empty bottles or notes in the house?
- History of depression/marital breakdown/bereavement?
- Previous self-poisoning or other suicide attempt?
- What treatment has *anyone* in the household been taking?
- Does patient have any other medical conditions (e.g. diabetes)?

Drugs commonly taken in self-poisoning

Drug (in descending order of frequency)	Toxic effect and dangers
Alcohol (often in combination with other drugs)	Vomiting, behaviour disturbance, drowsiness
Paracetamol (with or without dextropropoxyphene)	Liver failure several days after overdose (paracetamol alone). Coma, death within hours of overdose (combination with dextropropoxyphene — Co-proxamol)
Aspirin	Vomiting, hyperventilation, acidosis
Benzodiazepines (e.g. diazepam)	Drowsiness
Tricyclic or quadricyclic antidepressants	Convulsions, coma, ventricular fibrillation
Heroin (increasingly common in the young)	Coma, respiratory arrest

Further information about particular drugs or other substances may be obtained by telephoning a *Poisons Information Service* (number usually held in A & E office). If you do this be prepared to give: patient's name, age and sex, and details of any symptoms or problems already noted. You will be told about known effects, lethal dose, suggested treatment and antidotes.

Priority action
- Ask those accompanying patient to wait; they should not leave before being questioned
- Put patient in single room/cubicle if possible
- Explain to patient and relatives/friends that you want to prepare for examination and treatment.

Record:
- colour
- pulse
- blood pressure
- respirations
- pupil size and reaction to light
- level of consciousness.

When undressing the patient:
- search clothing for drugs/bottles/notes
- look for injuries (especially head and neck)

- look for needle marks (antecubital fossae, legs)
- look for skin pressure sores (in patients lying unconscious for long periods).

Talk to the patient
- Some will feign unconsciousness from unwillingness to admit what they have done, or from embarrassment
- Be friendly and non-judgmental in your approach
- Some patients repeatedly take overdoses and can be difficult and manipulative. Whilst being sympathetic do not get deeply involved. Refer such patients to the senior staff in the Department.

Treatment
This will depend on the time since the substance was ingested. Up to 4-6 hours after ingestion empty stomach by either:

An emetic   Ipecacuhana 30 ml + 1 litre water, or
Gastric lavage with a large-bore soft plastic tube.
Precautions: *Not* if gag reflex inhibited unless intubated
               Not if history of oesophageal varices or stomach ulcer
               Not if ingested petroleum distillates or corrosives.
Activated charcoal may be injected down the stomach tube to "adsorb" the poison.
Save gastric aspirate for toxicological analysis.

Other treatment
- milk and large quantities of fluid when corrosives have been taken
- supportive treatment:
  - i-v fluids, especially in salicylate poisoning
  - ventilation
  - anticonvulsants
- specific antidotes:
  - desferrioxamine via washout tube and i-v for iron poisoning
  - naloxone i-v for opiate poisoning or dextropropoxyphene overdose
  - acetylcysteine for paracetamol overdose.

Investigations
- blood salicylate level
- blood paracetamol level
- blood sugar
- urea and electrolytes
- urine for toxicology.

Carbon monoxide poisoning is often accidental but can be deliberate (self-gassing using car exhaust).

Symptoms:
— headache
— vomiting
— drowsiness

Signs:
— drowsiness/coma
— no hyperventilation
— cherry-red skin/mucosae

Treatment:
— 100% oxygen by endotracheal tube
— ventilation in severe cases
— hyperbaric oxygen in most severely poisoned.

Further management
• Social worker if problems at home, e.g. children unattended, elderly parents (see Appendix B)
• Psychiatric referral offered to all patients.

Transfer/discharge from A & E

Patient may be admitted to:
1. a general medical ward or ICU
2. a special drug overdose unit
3. a psychiatric unit if the overdose is not physically harmful, but the patient's mental state warrants inpatient management.

Patients may go home if:
— the family and GP are willing to cope
— there are not considered to be any significant physical or mental problems.

Remember: When dealing with enquiries from friends/relatives about the patient, confidentiality must be preserved.
---

8 Diabetic emergencies

These fall into two groups:
— **Hypo**glycaemia (low blood glucose)
— **Hyper**glycaemia (high blood glucose)
Hypoglycaemia and hyperglycaemia are immediately distinguished by simple blood glucose ("blood sugar") estimation. This should be performed immediately on arrival at A & E in all ill diabetic patients. Glucose oxidase reagent strips are used; one large drop of blood is required (see below).

HYPOGLYCAEMIA

* Can rapidly cause permanent brain damage
* *Unconsciousness is much more likely to be due to hypoglycaemia than to hyperglycaemia.* Insulin-treated patients are particularly at risk, but oral hypoglycaemic drugs can also cause hypoglycaemia.

Recognition
* the patient is usually a known diabetic reported to be well just before being brought to A & E
* the patient is often sweaty with dilated unequal pupils
* neurological or mental disturbance occurs, with confusion, aggression, coma, fits or a speech disorder
* paralysis of one or more limbs may occur
* "down-and-out" alcoholics who are not diabetic are also at risk of hypoglycaemia due to alcoholic liver damage. Their confused state may mimic drunkenness; they may be brought to A & E by the police
* small children who drink alcohol are also at risk of hypoglycaemia because the release of glycogen from the liver is inhibited.

Priority action
* **Airway;** care of the unconscious patient
* Reagent strip test for blood sugar:

— clean fingertip or earlobe with soap and water
— dry thoroughly
— do not use alcohol wipe (this alters the reading)
— squeeze large drop of blood onto glucose oxidase reagent
   strip
— time accurately and read quickly
— record the result
— a blood sample is simultaneously sent in a fluoride (yellow)
   tube to the laboratory for a more accurate glucose estimation.

Treatment given
• in unconscious or barely responsive patients 20-50 ml 50%
  dextrose by i-v injection (after blood has been taken for glucose
  measurement)
• milk and sandwiches when patient has regained consciousness.
Failure to respond immediately to these measures can mean:
• inadequate sugar replacement
• permanent brain damage due to prolonged hypoglycaemia
• another cause for impaired consciousness.
Further urgent measures to elevate blood sugar include:
• i-v — hydrocortisone
       — adrenaline
       — glucagon.

Transfer/discharge from A & E
Ward : For repeated episodes requiring stabilisation
          Patients suffering prolonged unconsciousness.
Home : Complete recovery from isolated episode.

Advice to patient on discharge
1. To help the patient avoid a further hypoglycaemic crisis, try to
   find out what brought on "hypo" attack, e.g.:
   • sudden exertion without adjustment of food and insulin
   • alcoholic binge
   • irregular eating pattern
   • stress, such as taking an exam.
   Reinforce the dangers of repeated hypo attacks.
2. Oral *glucose* or *sugar* should only be given in an emergency. A
   sandwich or milk and plain biscuits allow the blood sugar level to
   rise steadily rather than suddenly peaking.

HYPERGLYCAEMIA

This occurs when the blood glucose load is too high to be dealt
with by the body's insulin. It occurs if a diabetic:
— does not take treatment
— is injured

— develops an infection
— has a myocardial infarction.
Together with the rise in blood glucose there is usually an increase
in the acidity of the blood ("diabetic keto-acidosis"). The excess
glucose spills over from the blood into the urine, drawing water
with it, so increasing the volume of urine. Glucose and ketones
become detectable in the urine.

Recognition
* The blood sugar rises slowly so that symptoms develop over
  several hours or days
* Thirst and frequency of micturition are common
* Dehydration (dry tongue, sunken eyes, reduced skin turgor)
* Hyperventilation suggests ketoacidosis
* Drowsiness occurs often but coma is rare except in previously-
  undiagnosed elderly patients
* Symptoms often follow urinary, gastro-intestinal or respiratory
  infections.

Priority action
* Blood sugar
* Urea and electrolytes (renal failure can follow dehydration)
* Large volumes of i-v saline — this alone can lower blood sugar
  and improve clinical condition
* Potassium added to infusion after serum potassium level
  measured
* Insulin, i-v in small amounts, depending on blood sugar (may be
  delivered by continuous infusion pump)
* Sodium bicarbonate i-v if patient profoundly keto-acidotic (rarely
  required)
* Antibiotics i-v when evidence of infection present
* Blood sugar and serum potassium monitored frequently during
  early stages of treatment as both can fall rapidly to dangerously
  low levels.
* ECG (myocardial infarction?)
* Chest X-ray (chest infection?)
* Arterial blood gases and pH (acidity)
* Blood cultures (septicaemia?)
* Monitor:
  — pulse
  — blood pressure
  — conscious level
  — respiration
  — temperature.

Transfer from A & E
Admission to the ward is generally the rule for hyperglycaemic ill
patients.

9 Psychiatric emergencies

Many psychiatric emergencies are dealt with by doctors at the patient's home or at police stations, and so never come to A & E. Disturbed patients may come to hospital after:
— creating a public disturbance
— being found wandering on public property claiming depression, suicidal intent or loss of memory
— friends or relatives find they can no longer cope with the disturbed behaviour.

Abnormal behaviour or mental disturbance may be due to:
— physical disease (e.g. head injury, infection, dementia) ⎫ especially in the elderly
— side-effects of prescribed medication ⎬ ("toxic
— drug abuse confusional
— alcoholism ⎭ state")
— psychiatric disease (e.g. schizophrenia, depression)
— personality disorder
— attention-seeking.
It may be impossible immediately to identify the cause of abnormal behaviour.

Mentally disturbed patients may be:
— difficult or impossible to communicate with
— withdrawn, immobile or passive (mute, catatonic)
— violent, noisy and active (manic)
— suspicious, "hearing voices" (paranoid).

Priority action
• One experienced nurse should stay with patient
• Take to a quiet room away from other patients
• Remove valuable or dangerous objects from the room if patient is violent
• Don't attempt to reason; but listen to patient and give brief responses to indicate that you are listening
• Other staff should remain in close proximity

- A cigarette or a cup of coffee may be appropriate and calm the situation
- Drugs are normally used only as a last resort until a diagnosis is made
- Attempt to obtain details from relatives/attendants about:
  - past medical/psychiatric history
  - medications taken (e.g. treatment for Parkinson's Disease).

These may give clues to the diagnosis; it may be necessary to search the patient's clothing for medicine bottles and hospital appointment cards.

Transfer/discharge from A & E

- Most patients will return home in the care of family, GP and community psychiatric staff.
- Patients who are a danger to themselves or others are usually admitted to a psychiatric assessment unit.
- Patients with major physical disorders are admitted to general wards.

Some other aspects of the management of the mentally disturbed patient are dealt with in Appendix B—Social and legal problems.

10 Less common emergencies

SUSPECTED SERIOUS COMMUNICABLE DISEASE

Infectious diseases such as typhoid fever, infectious hepatitis, AIDS, meningococcal meningitis and poliomyelitis are extremely dangerous. They can be transmitted from one person to another by contact with infected body fluids or excreta. Extra care is required with AIDS because there is as yet no preventive vaccine or treatment.

There are two main considerations in the emergency management of these patients:
- care of patient including diagnostic investigations and urgent treatment
- protection of staff and other patients from infection. The patient is therefore nursed in isolation by the minimum number of personnel.

Recognition

Serious communicable disease is suspected in a pyrexial patient who has:
— come from a part of the world where such diseases are common (e.g. West or Central Africa)
— been in contact with people suffering, or at risk from, serious communicable disease (e.g. children from a school with an epidemic of meningococcal meningitis)
— diarrhoea
— jaundice (suggesting hepatitis)
— unexplained fever for five or more days
— drug addiction*
— haemophilia*
— history of homosexual activity*.

*risk factors for AIDS and hepatitis.

49

Priority action
- Barrier nursing (plastic apron, gowns and gloves) to protect staff and other patients
- Ensure porters, radiographers and other staff who come into contact with patient and soiled equipment are aware of infection risk
- Resuscitation with i-v fluids where necessary
- Avoid spillage of patient's excretions and secretions
- Wash hands after contact with patient
- Blood, urine, stool and swabs of all orifices are collected in sealed containers (labelled as infectious risk) and sent for urgent microbiological analysis
- AIDS and hepatitis B ("infectious hepatitis") — both are spread by contaminated blood; both are commoner among homosexuals and drug abusers
  Prevention of spread:
    - use gloves when handling patient
    - be extremely careful with needles and syringes
    - after needle-prick injury hepatitis B immunoglobulin is given as soon as possible (against hepatitis). There is currently no vaccine for AIDS
- Consider patient's psychological needs. He may be very frightened and will need support and reassurance.

Transfer of patient from A & E
Admission is invariably required, to:
1. side-room on general ward
2. Infectious Diseases Unit.
After transfer of patient either clean or dispose of all equipment according to local policy, e.g. rubbish for incineration and laundry in marked bags. All trolleys and surfaces cleaned with hypochlorite solution.

DROWNING

- Most victims are children or intoxicated adults
- Survival can occur up to 40 minutes after submersion even if no pulse is recordable at the onset of resuscitation. This is more likely in cold water drowning
- Cardiopulmonary resuscitation of drowned patients should therefore continue much longer than in cardiopulmonary arrests due to other causes.

Priority action

Resuscitation
- Cardiopulmonary resuscitation as described in Chapter 2
- Very slow re-warming as described for hypothermia (Chapter 5); too-rapid re-warming will increase cerebral oedema and cause brain damage
- Continued ventilation will improve blood oxygenation and reduce cerebral oedema
- I-v fluids are given to expand blood volume and improve circulation.

Record:
- pulse
- blood pressure
- respirations (if breathing spontaneously)
- conscious level
- pupil size.

Investigations
- arterial blood gases (P_aO_2 often low on breathing air)
- serum potassium (often reduced in drowning)
- serum sodium (increased in salt-water drowning)
- ECG (for arrythmias, especially ventricular fibrillation)
- chest X-ray.

Transfer from A & E
Patient usually admitted to ICU.

VASCULAR EMERGENCIES

Most patients with acute arterial problems already have diseased blood vessels (atherosclerosis), and:
- are usually elderly
- are often smokers
- may have had a previous stroke or heart attack
- may have other symptoms of narrowed arteries, e.g. chest pain (angina) or leg pain (claudication) on exercise.

The most common vascular emergencies are heart attacks (Chapter 3) and strokes (Chapter 5). The other vascular emergencies most likely to be seen in A & E are:

Arterial embolus in the leg. A clot and/or piece of diseased lining of the vessel wall is swept down the artery and blocks off the blood supply. Patient has sudden onset of pain with a white, *cold* leg. Pulses *cannot* be felt in the foot. Urgent operation required to remove the clot.

Deep vein thrombosis. Blood clot forms in the leg, commonly a few days after an operation, or after immobilisation, e.g. in plaster.

Patient has a *warm*, tender calf, and possibly oedema causing swelling of the foot and ankle. Pulses *can* be felt in the foot. If the clot breaks loose it can be carried to the lungs causing a *pulmonary embolus* which can be fatal. Priority action:
— venogram to establish the diagnosis
— admission to ward for i-v heparin to prevent further clotting.

Ruptured aortic aneurysm. Expansion of the aorta due to disease of its wall; rupture causes sudden abdominal pain (Chapter 6) and severe shock. Treatment is urgent operation. Mortality is 50%.

11 Ill children

Points to remember:

About the child:
- small children sicken rapidly; a happy boisterous child can become ill and prostrated within an hour
- children identify the source of their discomfort poorly and show the same responses (fever or vomiting) to many types of illness
- even an ill child fears outsiders. Fear and lack of self-control make many children cry when brought to hospital; inappropriate scolding can worsen this "bad behaviour". The help of parents is essential when calming such children; even their efforts may be unsuccessful. The child who willingly submits to being handled by strangers is truly ill.

About the parents:
- most parents become extremely anxious when their children become ill. Many people compensate for fear by anger, so some of the tensest situations in A & E involve the parents of ill children
- many children brought to A & E with medical problems come from families with severe social problems (see Appendix B).

Recognition of childhood illness

Fever and vomiting
- occur in many (especially infectious) conditions
- are non-specific signs of illness in children
- vomiting commonly follows a minor head injury (see Chapter 14).

Respiratory abnormalities
- rapid breathing is found in conditions affecting the lungs and trachea, and in diabetes, where the rapid respiration is an attempt to correct acidosis by blowing off CO_2. Even without these problems a febrile distressed child will breathe rapidly.

— prolonged wheezy expiration suggests asthma or an inhaled foreign body
— "grunting" occurs in small babies with pneumonia in an attempt to increase oxygen pressure in the lungs
— stridor ("whooping") on inspiration is a sign of croup, acute epiglottitis or a tracheal foreign body. Any of these can cause sudden, unexpected death, even in a child who appears quite well. *Never probe around in the mouth of a child with stridor — you could produce a critical obstruction to airflow.* The child should be kept as quiet and as comfortable as possible until the doctor arrives.

Abdominal symptoms
— vomiting and diarrhoea may occur in most suddenly-developing childhood illnesses as well as in abdominal disease, as in adults (see Chapter 6). Severe dehydration can develop in only a few hours.

Persistent crying
— indicates pain or discomfort; the cause is often an ear infection.

Management of the ill child (see also Chapter 21)
• Keep child and parents calm; use a side-room away from other ill or noisy patients
• Record:
   — temperature
   — respirations
   — pulse
• Investigations (according to condition):
   — chest X-ray (infection?)
   — full blood count, urea and electrolytes, blood sugar.

Poisoning in children
Accidental swallowing of tablets, berries, fungi and household substances are common causes for A & E attendance. Parents are often guilt-stricken or angry about what has happened.

Priority action
• the child should always be seen quickly
• try to ascertain what and how much has been taken
• record:
   — conscious level
   — pulse
   — respirations
   — pupil size
• note vomiting, abdominal pains
• don't force a reluctant toddler to be undressed

- provide a toy or other distraction: a torch is nearly always successful
- if an emetic is prescribed, the child will probably take it better from the mother — ask if a cup or spoon is more acceptable. Sometimes a syringe is the best way to get medicine between tightly clamped lips. Follow up with a drink — orange squash is usually more appreciated than water! This will increase the effect of the emetic.

Transfer/discharge from A & E

Home : Children not acutely ill with satisfactory home circumstances.
Ward : Any child whose condition may deteriorate
Any child in whom NAI is suspected (see Chapter 21)
Any child who has suffered a convulsion
Any child with respiratory difficulty
Any child with persistent diarrhoea and vomiting
Any child with raised temperature which does not settle with paracetamol.

Advice to parent on discharge

- Ensure child takes medication as prescribed
- Call GP or return to A & E if child's condition worsens.

PART 2

Injured patients

12 The injured patient in the Accident and Emergency Department

The common causes of injury bringing patients to A & E are:
Road Traffic Accidents (RTA's):
- — vehicle occupants
- — motorcyclists
- — pedestrians
- — bicyclists

Sports (e.g. football)
Industrial accidents
Domestic accidents
Fights, assault.

Usually, "major" injuries (e.g. fractured femur) will be brought in by ambulance, often with some warning of their arrival. "Minor" injuries (e.g. cut finger) usually arrive at A & E unannounced. But, remember, for the individual patient *his* or *her* injury is "major" to them, and requires equal consideration and care. The following stages of management apply to injured patients; the initials of each line make up the word

T R A U M A T I C

Triage — sorting patients into three broad categories by severity of injury and urgency of treatment required:
- • immediate (life-threatening)
- • urgent
- • can wait

Resuscitation and ***Registration***
Assessment
Undress
Medical examination and investigations
Analgesia
Treatment
Information
- — patient
- — relatives, friends
- — ward/GP

Clothing and valuables.

The following chapters look at the way various types of injury are managed in A & E, and the nurse's responsibilities.

Look for certain "patterns of injury":
Head and chest (RTAs)
Chest and abdomen (RTAs, sport)
Femur and tibia (motorcyclists, sport)
Cervical and thoracic spine (sports)
Hand fractures (fights)
Hand lacerations (industrial, domestic)
Spine, pelvis, heel (falls from a height)
Burns (industrial, domestic)
Face/jaw (fights, assault).

Some of these causes are commoner at characteristic times:

RTAs	— rush-hours, weekends, bank holidays
Sports injuries	— weekends (especially Saturday afternoons)
Fights, assaults	— late evening
Industrial accidents	— working hours.

When you see injured patients in A & E, think about **prevention**.
What factors contributed to this patient's accident?
Alcohol (top of the list by a long way, especially after 6 pm)
Carelessness on the road
Inadequate protection (seat-belts, crash-helmets, sports equipment)
Improper use of machinery
Children unsupervised in the home
Unsafe equipment at work or at home.

Anyone, at any time, can get caught up in the circumstances which inevitably lead to an injury. But there is definitely a tendency for some groups of people to attend A & E more often than would be expected by chance. The glib term "accident-prone" for these habitual attenders is meaningless. Accidents are *caused*; habitual attenders show unstable behaviour patterns, with excessive risk-taking, carelessness with recognised precautions, plain thoughtlessness, and often a background of alcohol abuse and/or social deprivation (broken home, marital discord, unemployment, mental illness, prison, etc.).

Society's underprivileged account for more A & E trauma patients than those with the advantages of a job, a home, and financial security.

13 Multiple injuries

Recognition
Severe injuries to two or more systems (e.g. chest and head; abdomen and limbs)
Often life-threatening
Require urgent resuscitation.

Common causes
Road traffic accidents, especially motorcyclists and unrestrained rear-seat car passengers
Falls from a height.

Assessment
The first priority is the airway. Asphyxia is the commonest cause of death after an accident. A patient who has been rescued from an accident should never die of an obstructed airway in A & E.

The first assessment is therefore of the *patient's ability to breathe spontaneously without obstruction.* Signs of airway obstruction to look for are:
— laboured breathing (dyspnoea)
— bluish tinge to face and lips, with warm skin (cyanosis)
— deteriorating consciousness.
Common causes of airway obstruction to look for are:
— loss of consciousness (head injury), which may lead to:
  — tongue falling back
  — dislodged false teeth
  — inhaled vomit or secretions (from nose, trachea, bronchi)
— oedema of pharynx and larynx (especially in facial and neck injuries)
— bleeding into the pharynx.

Immediate action
Place patient semi-prone, protecting neck
Apply suction
Remove teeth/foreign matter from mouth
Ensure doctor alerted urgently

The patient is then prepared for a preliminary assessment of his injuries.

Look at:
— position patient is lying in
— shape of limbs
— damage to clothing, bleeding

Ask the conscious patient:
— what hurts?
— can he move fingers/toes?

Undress the patient:
— two nurses required
— unzip and unbutton first
— ease off clothes, uninjured side first
— if clothing tight, cut off (along seams if possible)
— retain cut off clothing.

	Look for
• head injury?	conscious level; bleeding from scalp, nose, ears
• chest injury?	respiration; external signs of injury
• spinal injury?	movements and sensation in limbs; local bruising
• abdominal or pelvic injury?	marks on skin; blood at urinary meatus
• limb fractures or dislocations?	deformities, swelling, localised pain.

Assess conscious level (Chapter 14 — make sure you know how this is done: it is very important).

Start recording pulse, blood pressure, respiration.

Look for signs of blood loss:
• Pallor
• Sweating
• Thirst
• Rapid pulse
• Low blood pressure.

Approximate blood loss is estimated as:

	units of blood (1 unit = approx. 500 ml)
Fractured femur*	4
Fractured tibia*	1-2
Upper limb fractures*	1
Chest injury	100 ml per rib fracture
Abdominal injury	4
Pelvic injury	2-6
Head injury	1
Open wounds	variable

Urgent action — trauma resuscitation
There are clear priorities here, although several components of the immediate treatment of severe injuries are performed simultaneously rather than in sequence.

Priorities
1. **Airway** (remove obstruction; suction; Guedel airway; sometimes endotracheal tube; rarely tracheostomy).
2. **I-v infusion** (usually two sites; central vein if peripheral veins collapsed). Haemaccel or other plasma expander is given while awaiting blood. A bacterial filter and blood warmer are used if more than 4 units are to be transfused. In dire emergency Group O rhesus negative (universally compatible) blood is used. *Commence record of fluid given.*
3. **Insertion of chest drain** (to relieve pneumothorax) — see Chapters 4 and 15. Any open chest wounds are covered.
4. **Blood sample** taken for haemoglobin, haematocrit, urea and electrolytes, and grouping and cross-matching. Laboratory must be alerted to ensure urgent testing. If patient unidentified ensure registration number is clearly marked on the sample and laboratory request card.
5. **Open fractures** and other wounds covered with sterile dressings. *Direct pressure* to control bleeding.
6. **Neurological observations** started if head injury, and **girth measurements** if abdominal injury suspected.
7. **Oxygen** by mask (24-28%).
8. **Stabilisation** of obvious long bone fractures temporarily with emergency splint or plaster back-slab; Thomas splint for femoral fractures (see Chapters 17 and 22).
9. **Central venous pressure** line inserted to estimate circulating volume.
10. **Naso-gastric tube** passed, especially if stomach full — danger of aspiration of vomit.
11. **Peritoneal lavage** (see Chapter 16) may be required.
12. **Pain relief** — if no head injury:
     - "Entonox" (see Appendix A)
     - pethidine + anti-emetic
     - papaveretum + anti-emetic
    — if patient has had head injury:
     - codeine phosphate.
13. **Further information** from patient/relatives/G.P.:
     - relevant medical history (diabetes, heart disease, asthma, epilepsy, alcohol problems)

---

*more if compound ("open") fractures

- regular drugs (especially steroids, insulin)
- allergies (e.g. penicillin)
- tetanus immunity.

14. **Antibiotics** for open wounds and fractures.
15. **Antitetanus toxoid** (ATT) —easy to forget in the heat of the moment.
16. **Urinary Catheter** — measure output.
17. **Urine Specimens** tested for blood (pelvic injury?), glucose (diabetes?) and protein (kidney injury?).
18. **Relatives informed** of patient's condition and proposed immediate treatment (e.g. operation), either by phone or preferably in person.
19. **Patient's clothing and valuables** must be labelled and bagged. Local policy followed for recording and safe-keeping.

A lot is happening at once in the immediate management of a multiply injured patient. **Accurage records** are essential, especially of:

— conscious level
— pulse, blood pressure, respiration, temperature
— fluids given (types and volumes)
— drugs given (times and doses)
— urine output
— specimens sent to laboratory.

Transfer from A & E

Usually: • directly to theatre
- to ICU (e.g. for ventilation)
- to theatre via the ward
- to the ward.

Major disasters

These are uncommon. The term means a situation in which more patients are admitted at once than the hospital's system can cope with normally. All larger hospitals have a Major Disaster Plan which lays down the organisation for action in these circumstances. You should look at this document while you are working in A & E. Occasional unannounced "rehearsals" of the Plan are carried out. The arrangements include:

- *special call-out* system following alert
- *triage* — sorting patients by severity of injury and urgency of treatment required
- *transfer or discharge* of other patients to make room for new admissions to the wards
- *change in use of rooms* in A & E, outpatients, etc. to make room for casualties and their treatment
- *communication* between hospital staff and patients, relatives, police and the media; and between A & E and theatre, wards, ICU, X-ray, the pathology departments and the blood bank.

14 Head injuries

This is the commonest cause of death in people aged between 15 and 24. Every year one person in 50 attends an A & E department with a head injury. Half are under 30, and after 6 p.m. many are drunk.

Recognition

Altered consciousness, varying from a transient loss of consciousness ("concussion" — an imprecise term best avoided) to major brain injury with complete unresponsiveness to external stimuli.

Wounds of the scalp and face, with or without loss of consciousness. These bleed freely often leading to exaggerated estimates of blood loss.

Important features in the patient's immediate history include:
- nature of injury (direct blow — fracture likely; rapid deceleration — diffuse brain injury)
- length of post-traumatic amnesia (PTA): memory loss for events after the injury
- vomiting (common after head injury, especially in children)
- fits (serious sign of local brain injury)
- other injuries (e.g. chest).

Causes
- Road traffic accidents, including pedestrians
- Falls
- Assaults and fights
- Sports.

Assessment

The *level of consciousness* is the fundamental estimate of brain function and is recorded on a scale ("coma scale") usually printed on a "Head Injury Observation Chart". The following responses are recorded. **These are very important.**

Eye opening
(note if eyes closed by
swelling)
— spontaneous; sleep/wake rhythms
— to speech (not necessarily a command)
— to pain (applied to limbs)
— no response.

Best verbal response
(note if endotracheal
tube or tracheostomy
— orientated in time and place
— confused conversation, disorientated
— inappropriate speech (intelligible but
  random words)
— incomprehensible (jargon, gibberish)
— no speech.

Best motor response
(usually record the
better arm response;
note if spinal injury
or limb fractures
present)
— obeys commands
— localising response (attempts to
  remove pain agent)
— flexes to painful stimulus: rapid or slow,
  but with purpose
— extends to painful stimulus:
  "decerebrate rigidity" (indicates severe
  brain injury).

Pupil size and reaction
   Pupil size: the extremes — very dilated or very constricted ("pin-point" — may be due to drugs), are obvious, but anywhere in between *can* be normal. Record by drawings: the observation chart may have a pupil size scale in millimetres for guidance. Look for:

**Change in size over time
Difference between the two eyes**

   Pupil reaction (normal is a brisk constriction); test with the room lights off and a torch with a good battery shone briefly in each eye in turn.

Limb movements
Test and record each arm and each leg:
— normal power
— mild weakness
— severe weakness
— spastic flexion
— extension
— no response.

Vital signs
— pulse
— blood pressure
— respirations
— temperature.
   Rising pulse and falling blood pressure suggest raised intracranial pressure (e.g. due to brain swelling).

Increased respirations may be due to lung collapse or aspiration pneumonia (the commonest cause of death in patients with otherwise uncomplicated head injury). Major changes in respiratory rate may indicate damage to the "respiratory centre" in the brain.

Low temperature may be found in patients who have been lying unconscious out-of-doors in the colder months (see Chapter 5). Rectal temperatures are more accurate and safer than oral.

Other features
Record:
— fits (type, number, side)
— incontinence
— drugs given.

Remember
- *Change* is important, especially in level of consciousness, so the observations need to be repeated regularly, usually every 15 minutes in A & E.
- *One nurse* should make the observations as she will notice changes more quickly. If you hand over for a meal break or shift change make a joint observation with the person who takes over.
- *Alcohol* or *drugs* can obscure all the above observations, so extra care is needed with patients known or believed to have taken either.

General examination
- Other injuries, especially neck injury which can easily be missed in an unconscious patient.
- Also look for watery discharge, indicating CSF leaks, from the nose or ears (a sign of fracture of the base of the skull).

Other investigations
- Skull X-ray (for fractures, but their absence does not exclude a life-threatening complication)
- Cervical spine X-ray (to exclude neck injury in an unconscious patient)
- Chest X-ray (associated chest injury is common and worsens the patient's condition)
- CT (computed tomography) scan. The best means of diagnosing an intracranial clot (extradural or subdural haematoma), but only available in major centres.
- Haemoglobin, urea and electrolytes.

Priority action for patients with major head injuries
- **Ensure airway is unobstructed**
- The scalp will be cleaned, shaved and lacerations sutured
- Antibiotics for compound skull fractures, including patients with CSF leaks from nose or ears

- ATT if wound present
- I-v infusion in unconscious patient
- Naso-gastric tube to prevent aspiration of stomach contents
- Urinary catheter in unconscious patient.

Transfer/discharge from A & E

Home : Only for very minor head injuries with no skull fracture, fully conscious and orientated, and stable observations. Admission policies vary. Patient is discharged only if a responsible adult is present at home to look after patient.

Ward : For observation, usually overnight.

ICU : For severe head injuries, especially with chest problems. Ventilation may be required to reduce cerebral oedema.

Theatre : For suture of large lacerations, or if other injuries require surgery, or for urgent decompression of intracranial clot.

Neurosurgical : For CT scan and operation to evacuate clot,
unit elevate a depressed fracture, or for treatment of penetrating injuries (e.g. gun-shot wounds).

Maxillo-facial (or plastic surgery) unit — For severe facial injuries (usually of lesser urgency than other major injuries).

Eye Unit — For severe eye injuries. The simple "black eye" (a haematoma in the soft tissues around the eye) is treated with chloramphenicol eye ointment to prevent infection, and a pad.

Instructions to patients on discharge (immediately, or after a period of observation)

For 2-3 days following injury:

- Rest
- Do not return to work
- Do not drive or operate machinery
- Do not drink alcohol
- Take simple pain-killers (e.g. paracetamol) for headache
- Return to hospital if severe headache, visual disturbance, drowsiness or repeated vomiting occur.

Most patients who return to hospital with post-head injury symptoms have failed to observe the above advice.

15 Chest injuries

These range from the single rib fracture to major life-threatening injuries, often associated with other trauma.

Recognition
- Pain in the chest following trauma
- Difficulty with breathing (dyspnoea)
- Coughing up blood (haemoptysis)
- Signs of blood loss (sweating, pallor, rapid pulse, low blood-pressure)
- Sometimes associated with other injuries (e.g. abdomen, pelvis, head).

Common causes
Contact sports (especially rugby)
Road traffic accidents
Assault
Industrial/agricultural injuries
Falls in the elderly.

Assessment
- **Airway unobstructed?**
- Any open chest wound?
- Chest movements — look for *flail chest*: a segment of the chest wall moves *in* on inspiration and *out* on expiration ("paradoxical respiration"). This is a serious condition due to multiple fractures of several ribs
- Signs of respiratory distress; cyanosis?
- Marks on chest wall, e.g. imprint of clothing or seat-belt; local bruising
- Local tenderness, may be due to rib fractures
- Respirations
- Surgical emphysema — crackling sensation under the skin caused by air in the tissues
- Signs of blood loss
- Other injuries

- Relevant history (e.g. asthma, bronchitis, smoking); regular medicines.

Investigations
- Chest X-ray (50% of rib fractures may not show up on an X-ray)
- Haemoglobin
- Arterial blood sample (usually from femoral artery) for oxygen tension measurement ("blood gases")
- ECG (if sternum fractured, or other reason to suspect injury to heart or great vessels)
- Blood cross-matched (for major or open chest injuries).

Priority action
This is directed at:
- providing adequate ventilation
- restoring blood volume
- avoiding infection.
Priorities are therefore:
1. Adequate unobstructed airway.
2. Chest drain for patients with chest wounds or flail chest, or if blood has collected in the chest (*haemothorax*) (see Chapter 4).
3. Closure of any open wound (which could act as a valve, allowing air into the chest causing a *tension pneumothorax* and suffocation), with a sterile air-tight dressing.
4. I-v infusion.
5. Antibiotics.
6. Pain relief (oral analgesia or local or regional anaesthesia — see Appendix A). Most analgesics depress respiration and the cough reflex, especially opiates, pethidine and codeine, and these should be avoided. Paracetamol is safer.
7. Treat other injuries.

Transfer/discharge from A & E
Home   : For minor chest injuries without compromised respiration.
Ward   : For observation, repeat X-ray and blood gas measurement, pain control and chest physiotherapy.
ICU   : — if endotracheal intubation and assisted ventilation required (e.g. for multiple rib fractures with flail segment)
          — patients with bilateral chest drains.
Theatre : — for thoracotomy in uncontrollable bleeding
          — if injury to trachea, major bronchi, heart or aorta
          — for treatment of other injuries.

Advice to patient on discharge
- Pain inhibits deep breathing; this leads to accumulation of secretions in the lungs and the danger of infection (pneumonia)

- Take pain-killers in prescribed dose to allow comfortable deep breathing
- Try to maintain normal level of physical activity rather than retiring to bed
- *No smoking*
- Do *not* bandage or bind up bruised or broken ribs
- If cough develops or pain increases, contact GP.

16 Abdominal and pelvic injuries

These injuries are "hidden from view" (unlike, for example a fractured tibia), so are diagnosed indirectly and may be missed initially.

Recognition
- Abdominal pain following an accident
- Haematuria
- Signs of hypovolaemic shock not explained by "visible" injuries (e.g. fractured femur)
- Penetrating injury (e.g. stab wound).

Common causes
- High-speed road traffic accidents
- Contact sports
- Falls from a height.

Assessment
- Blunt or penetrating injury?
- Pulse and blood pressure
- External signs of injury:
  — bruising
  — imprint of clothing or seat-belt on skin
  — discolouration of skin (sign of urine tracking under the skin in bladder rupture)
  — blood at urinary meatus (urethral or bladder injury)
- Localised tenderness:
  — lower ribs: liver or spleen injury?
  — pelvis: fracture, or bladder or urethral injury?
  — loin: kidney injury?
- Pain in shoulder-tip (especially if patient head-down) suggests blood in the peritoneal cavity (irritation of diaphragm, which has the same nerve supply as the shoulder-tip)
- Girth measurements. Sometimes used to estimate increase in abdominal size (e.g. with bleeding)
- Peritoneal lavage. The bladder is emptied via a urinary catheter,

then 1-2 litres of normal saline are injected into the peritoneal
cavity through a peritoneal dialysis catheter (introduced under
local anaesthesia). The fluid is then drained by gravity — the
giving set is placed below the patient and allowed to refill — and
inspected for blood, bile, urine or intestinal contents
* Other injuries: chest? head?

Investigations
* Test urine for blood, protein (urinary tract injury?)
* Haemoglobin (for base-line)
* Haematocrit (more immediate indicator of blood loss than
  haemoglobin level)
* Abdominal X-ray (abnormal gas, fluid or tissue shadows
  suggesting organ damage)
* Pelvis X-ray (fractures?)
* Chest X-ray (lower rib fractures suggest liver or spleen injury)
* Intravenous pyelogram (IVP) and/or urethrogram if urinary tract
  injury suspected
* Blood cross-matched if signs of blood loss, or if surgery likely.

Priority action
* I-v drip (saline if not shocked: Haemaccel if signs of blood loss)
* Naso-gastric tube
* Urinary catheter (suprapublic if urethral injury suspected)
* Open wounds are covered with occlusive dressing
* *No* attempt is made to remove any penetrating object in A & E
  — catastrophic bleeding may occur
* Analgesia is given with caution so as not to mask important
  physical signs.

Transfer/discharge from A & E
Ward   : Most patients with abdominal injuries require admission
             for observation; the diagnosis of e.g. ruptured spleen may
             not be apparent for several hours and depends on the
             surgeon observing *change* in the patient's condition.
             Pelvic injuries (e.g. fractures) need admission for
             analgesia, sometimes traction, and blood transfusion.
Theatre : Severe injuries with persistent hypotension and rapid
             pulse require urgent laparotomy to control bleeding
             Penetrating injuries, for exploration
             Urethral injuries, for repair
             Occasionally, some pelvic fractures.
ICU   : Multiply injured patients.
Home   : Only for minor injuries, e.g. avulsion pelvic fractures (piece
             of bone pulled off by muscle action, usually in
             sportsmen).

Advice to patient on discharge
Rest with adequate analgesics: avoid constipation (common with
 codeine and derivatives). Take plenty of fluids, fibre and fruit.
Return to A & E if pain getting worse rather than better.
Return to A & E if haematuria develops.

17 Limb injuries

Most A & E attendances are for limb injuries. Damage to soft tissues, including nerves, blood vessels and tendons, is just as important as fractures and dislocations. Infections, usually of the hand, are also common and can be serious.

Fractures are either *open* ("compound", i.e. the skin is broken over the bone, thus with danger of infection), or *closed* (with intact overlying skin). If a fracture involves a *joint* it is more serious, as arthritis may develop later unless the fragments are accurately repositioned.

Most fractures which are *displaced* (i.e. the bones are out of alignment) require *reduction* (replacement in the normal alignment), as do all *dislocations* (with very few exceptions). Reduction often requires a GA, and therefore usually admission, although some reductions can be done in A & E under regional anaesthesia (see Appendix A). The corrected position is then held with plaster of Paris or other external splintage (see Chapter 22). Sometimes, especially if a joint is involved, an operation is required to hold the reduction by *internal fixation* (plates and screws), or *traction* may be used.

Upper limb injuries are more common than lower limb injuries; hand injuries alone account for up to one quarter of all A & E trauma attendances. Socially and economically (because of time lost from work) they are among the most important injuries treated in the Department.

Common causes
Upper limb:
  Accidents at work (lacerations, crush injuries, amputations). One-third of all industrial injuries are to the hand
  Accidents in the home and garden (lacerations and penetrating injuries)
  Falls (fractures, especially the lower end of the radius in the elderly, often women — Colles' fracture; and in children — "greenstick fracture": a growing bone is less brittle than an adult bone).

Lower limb:
    Motorcycle accidents (especially fractured femur)
    Football (especially knee, tibia and ankle injuries)
    Pedestrians struck by vehicle (tibial fractures)
    Falls from a height (heel fractures)
    Falls in the elderly (fractured neck of femur).

Recognition
- Pain and swelling
- Loss of function (e.g. elderly woman unable to walk after a fall: fractured neck of femur; footballer unable to straighten knee after twisting injury: torn cartilage)
- Deformity (fracture or dislocation)
- Wound, with or without loss of movement or feeling
- Crush injury
- Amputation.

Assessment
- Other injuries?
- Patient's general condition (pulse, blood pressure)
- When and where did injury occur?
- Check circulation and sensation in the limb beyond the injury. Note that movement may be inhibited by pain
- Deformity?
- Wound?
- Swelling?
- Self-inflicted? Look for evidence of previous wounds, usually multiple superficial slashes on the front of the wrist
- When did patient last eat or drink? (For timing of GA).

Investigations
- X-ray (if fracture, dislocation or foreign body suspected)
- Haemoglobin and cross-match (for major limb fractures, or if operation planned)
- Chest X-ray (if patient over 50 and requiring GA)
- ECG (as for chest X-ray)
- Pus swab to bacteriology laboratory (*before* giving antibiotics) if any discharge present, e.g. from abscess.

Priority action
- Carefully remove all clothing from area of injury, if necessary by cutting
- Immobilise obvious fractures temporarily (emergency splint or plaster backslab) to reduce pain and bleeding, and prevent further displacement
- Remove rings and bracelets
- Cover open wounds with sterile dressing

- Apply local pressure, which stops nearly all bleeding; there is *no place* for tourniquets in A & E (except in theatre)
- Elevate limb:
    leg - raise foot of trolley
    arm and hand - on pillows and/or a sling
- I-v infusion for major injuries
- Antibiotics for open fractures and large or contaminated wounds
- ATT if wound present and patient not immune
- Pain relief — Entonox initially (patient-controlled, thus safe), then if severe pain pethidine or papaveretum if not contra-indicated by head, chest or abdominal injury (see Chapters 14,15,16).

Treatment
Most limb injuries are treated in A & E and discharged home.

Suturing
Small clean lacerations are sutured under local anaesthetic.
Superficial cuts, or those on delicate skin (e.g. the eyelids or shins) can be held with skin closure strips.

Reduction of fractures and dislocations

Shoulder dislocations	— reduced under sedation or GA; sling and body bandage applied to prevent re-dislocation
Forearm fractures	— reduced and plaster applied (see Chapter 22) under GA or regional anaesthesia
	— occasionally local anaesthetic solution may be injected into the fracture site
Hand and finger fractures and dislocations	— reduced under regional anaesthesia; bandaging (see below) or plaster slab applied
Major limb fractures and dislocations (e.g. tibia)	— usually need admission and a GA.

Aspiration of joint
Usually the knee after a sports injury. A sterile procedure, followed by application of a compression bandage (see Chapter 22).

Bandaging (See also Chapter 22)
Sprains/soft tissue injuries (and some fractures — crepe or elastic tubular bandage, with sling for elevation.
Toe/undisplaced finger fractures — strapped to neighbouring uninjured digit for support.
Clavicle — sling, sometimes with figure-of-eight bandage over shoulder with padding over fracture site.

Plaster (See also Chapter 22)
Undisplaced fractures, and some others (e.g. humerus, scaphoid,
metatarsals) do not require reduction, but need immobilisation for
comfort and to allow healing. Plaster is also used to support some
soft-tissue injuries (e.g. severe ankle sprains), and to protect
wounds which have been sutured.

Incision and drainage
— Superficial abscesses (e.g. paronychia) — drained in A & E under
  regional anaesthesia
— Major infections - admission and GA
— Sub-ungual haematoma (bleeding under a nail) - released by
  piercing the nail with a heated paper clip - dramatic relief of
  pain!

Transfer/discharge from A & E
Home   : The majority of patients with limb injuries are not
            admitted. Advice on discharge (see below) is essential for
            all patients. Patients on crutches must be taught to use
            them safely before discharge.
Ward   : Patients for whom immediate discharge may be unsuitable
            or impracticable, e.g.:
            • reduction of fracture, or other injury, where much
              swelling is expected
            • when regular observation of circulation is required (e.g.
              supracondylar fractures in children)
            • open fractures
            • late at night
            • unsuitable home conditions
            • the elderly
            • inability to manage crutches
            • infections requiring i-v antibiotics
            • waiting for operation
            • self-inflicted injuries, which require psychiatric referral.
            The ward should be informed in advance by A & E if any
            special equipment is required, e.g. special bed, traction
            apparatus.
Theatre : • Fractures for reduction or operation
            • Large lacerations, especially if contaminated
            • Major infections, for drainage
            • If required for other injuries.

Advice to patient on discharge
Specific advice to patients with plasters is given in Chapter 22.
• Any injured limb must be *elevated*: the arm in a sling; and the leg
  at least at hip level. (A footrest or stool is not high enough to
  keep down swelling). The foot of the bed should be raised at
  night.

- Exercise all unsplinted parts of the limb to avoid stiffness.
- If fingers or toes become blue or numb, return to A & E at once.
- Take analgesics regularly to control pain in the first 48 hours.
- If pain worsens rather than improves, return to A & E.
- Do not remove dressings or splintage before the time advised.
- Support bandages may be removed for washing.
- If prescribed antibiotics take full course.
- Attend GP's Surgery or A & E for removal of sutures as directed.

18 Spinal injuries

The most important consideration here is *damage to the spinal cord*. This occurs only in a small proportion of spinal injuries, but produces devastating results:
— *paraplegia* (loss of function of the lower half of the body - thoracic and lumbar injuries)
— *quadruplegia* (loss of function of all four limbs - cervical injuries).
About a thousand of these injuries occur each year in Britain. Most patients are young and otherwise fit, and often active sports people.

Recognition
- Pain in the spine following an injury
- Inability to move arms or legs
- Altered sensation in the limbs
- Sudden onset of low back pain following lifting or other strenuous activity (sometimes with sciatica — pain down one leg)
- Gunshot wounds or stabbing injuries to the back or neck.

Any patient unconscious from a head injury must be suspected of having a spinal injury.

Common causes
- Falls, especially from horses
- Diving (shallow water)
- Rugby (neck injury in the scrum or a tackle)
- RTAs, especially motorcyclists
- Industrial accidents (mining, construction work).

Assessment
In any patient with a spinal injury the main concern is to *avoid causing further damage to the spinal cord*. This can happen by moving a patient roughly, or bending his neck or back, which could convert a partial into a complete division of the cord, if there is an unrecognised fracture or dislocation.

- Airway secure?
- Respiration. (Cord injury in the neck results in paralysis of the intercostal muscles and sometimes the diaphragm)
- Any other injuries? Head injury?
- Ability to move all four limbs
- Sensation in all four limbs
- Bladder full? (Lack of sensation and motor power to void urine)
- Priapism? (Persistent erection, due to disturbance of pelvic nerves).

Priority action
- Ensure radio-translucent mattress/trolley available
- Do not move patient without medical supervision
- Two nurses must undress patient. Clothes should be loosened; close-fitting garments will need to be cut off (preferably along seams)
- Support head and neck with sandbags or temporary collar
- Record pulse, blood pressure (may be low due to "spinal shock" — gut blood vessels dilate due to damage to their nerve supply)
- Patient is examined for external signs of spinal injury (bruising, swelling, local tenderness)
- Patient is *log-rolled* (3-4 people required) to examine the back
- If airway obstruction/vomiting occurs patient should be log-rolled onto his side. Suction must be immediately available
- Stay with patient and tell him what is happening — he will be lying flat, unable to see anything, and probably very frightened
- When transporting patient to X-ray ensure porters have been warned to avoid uneven floor surfaces.

Investigations
- X-ray (spine, chest)
- Urine test (blood, sugar, protein)
- Haemoglobin
- Cross-match
- Urea and electrolytes.

Emergency treatment may be summarised as:

> **Resuscitation**
> **Prevent complications**
> **Pain relief**

Resuscitation
- Airway
- I-v fluids
- Care of the paralysed patient (see also Chapter 5).

Prevent complications
- Prevent further cord damage:
  - stabilise neck with sandbags
  - move patient by log-rolling only
  - "halter" traction (sling under the chin) sometimes used for neck injuries, or a temporary collar
- Prevent pressure sores — these can start developing in an hour:
  - make *absolutely sure* the patient is not lying on a wrinkled sheet or canvas, or on any projection or hard object
  - turn regularly as directed
  - if cord injury strongly suspected or confirmed, patient may be transferred to a special turning bed (Stoke Mandeville bed) or frame (Stryker frame)
- Prevent urinary infection:
  - if cord injury confirmed, catheterise under sterile conditions. Send CSU.

Pain relief
Once the spine is stabilised, pain is reduced, and in cord injury is usually absent below the level of damage (despite other injuries — e.g. limb fractures). Mild analgesics probably suffice. The patient is likely to be frightened, and needs reassurance.

Transfer/discharge from A & E

Theatre : For insertion of skull traction device ("halo" or "Crutchfield tongs") in cervical injuries, or for treatment of other injuries. In established spinal cord injury operation (other than to reduce dislocations) is of no benefit: the structure of the cord is too complex for repair.

Ward : For spinal injuries without cord damage, usually for analgesia and bedrest, and a collar for neck injuries (e.g. "whiplash injury" in a car accident). Acute low back pain may require skin traction (5 lb(2 kg) each leg), and sedation to relax muscle spasm.

Transfer : To Regional Spinal Injuries Centre for paraplegic and quadruplegic patients, by ambulance or helicopter with a nurse escort.

Home : Only for patients with minor spinal injuries with no neurological abnormality, and ability to pass urine and to sit and stand comfortably. A ready-made corset or plaster of Paris jacket may be prescribed.

The relatives of a patient with a spinal cord injury are very anxious and require information. Within the first 24 hours the outcome can never be 100% certain; however total paralysis and loss of sensation present from the moment of the accident rarely recover.

Advice to patient on discharge

- Rest in bed on firm mattress.
- Take regular pain-killers.
- If collar prescribed, wear this all the time (except for washing) until clinic follow-up.
- Avoid constipation: pain-killers and bedrest combine to cause this and increase discomfort.
- Drink plenty of fluids.
- Do simple exercises (bending back forwards, sideways and in rotation) for low back pain after acute symptoms have subsided.
- Do not stoop.
- Lift by bending at the knees, keeping back straight.
- Out-patient physiotherapy may be arranged.
- Return to A & E if:
  - pain becomes much more severe
  - weakness in arms or legs develops
  - tingling, numbness or pins and needles in arms or legs develops
  - bowel or urinary disturbance develops.

19 Burns

Burns are frightening, to the patient and sometimes to the nurse as well. Calmness and reassurance are essential. The two major risks of burns are:

> **Fluid loss**
> **Infection**

Extensive burns are often relatively painless due to destroyed nerve endings in the skin. *But these patients are much more ill than they seem.*

Recognition
There is usually a clear history of the injury, including the cause.

Causes
- Dry heat (flames, explosions, sunshine)
- Scalds (boiling water or other liquids)
- Chemicals (acids, corrosives)
- Tar and bitumen
- Molten metal
- Electricity
- Friction (e.g. "road burns")
- Lightning, radiation (rare).

Never forget the possibility of non-accidental injury (see Chapter 21) in children with scalds, especially of the feet and buttocks, or cigarette burns.

Assessment
- **Airway** (at risk in burns of the face and neck due to oedema, which can develop very rapidly)
- Note *time* of burn, to estimate amount of fluid lost by the time patient reaches A & E
- Note *cause* of burn: any chemical or corrosive still on skin? (If so, flood immediately with cold tap-water)
- Pulse, blood pressure, respirations

- Any special areas involved?
  - hands
  - eyelids
  - ears
  - circumferential burns of limbs
- Inhalation of smoke, hot air or chemical fumes?
- Other injuries?
- Area* of burn is estimated. This will help to assess the volume of fluid lost which requires replacement
- Depth of burn is estimated:
  - "partial thickness": growing layer of skin (dermis) is intact and burn will heal
  - "full thickness": dermis is destroyed; skin-graft will be required to avoid contracture and deformity

Often the burn is a mixture of partial and full thickness: the initial treatment (see below) is however the same for both types

- Note patient's *age*
- Ask patient his *weight*, or estimate it.

The chances of a patient dying from a burn depend on:
  - the *area* (the larger the more likely)
  - the patient's *age* (extremes of age are more vulnerable
  - the *depth* of the burn (full thickness burns are twice as likely to cause death as partial thickness burns of the same area).

Priority action
The burned patient often looks deceptively well on arrival. The effects of fluid loss (depletion of water, sodium and protein) take several hours to appear.

- **Ensure secure airway in burns of face or neck** (intubation or tracheostomy may be necessary)
- Wash off any chemical or corrosive on skin with copious cold water
- Remove clothing except where adherent to burned area
- Cover burn with wet sterile pads, for comfort and to prevent infection
- I-v fluids are given for burns of over 10% in children or 15% in adults (this guideline may vary in different hospitals). In major burns (over 30%) two i-v infusions may be required. Haemaccel and plasma are given to replace fluid loss from burned surface.

---

*The quick guide is the "Rule of Nines":

Head and neck — 9%	Front of lower limb — 9%
Each upper limb — 9%	Back of lower limb — 9%
Front of trunk — 2 × 9% (18%)	Back of trunk — 2 × 9% (18%)
Perineum — 1%	

In babies the head is relatively larger (15%) and lower limbs smaller than in adults.

For full thickness burns blood is required to replace destroyed red cells.

The fluid volumes given and the rate of infusion are calculated from the *area burned*, the *length of time since* the burn and the *patient's weight*. Fluid loss is the main early cause of death in patients with major burns

- In burns of over 10% blood is taken for:
  - haematocrit (packed cell volume, measure of the 'concentration' of the blood, and the most accurate estimate of fluid lost)
  - haemoglobin
  - urea and electrolytes
  - cross-match (for full-thickness burns over 10%)
- Pain relief:
  - small frequent doses of i-v morphine for severe burns
  - i-m pethidine for less extensive burns
- Anti-emetic to control nausea
- Naso-gastric tube if face or neck burned
- Unless immediate surgery is planned, or burn affects face or throat, encourage patient to drink, especially if i-v fluids are not being given
- Oxygen by mask, if smoke inhaled. These patients will also require a chest X-ray and arterial blood gas estimation
- Check tetanus immunity
- Swabs from burned area, adjacent skin, nose, throat and perineum (most infections which develop in burns come from the patient's own body)
- Urinary catheter in major burns, to measure urine output and obtain CSU
- Aspirate large blisters under sterile conditions
- Elevate burned limbs to reduce swelling
- Clean and dress burns (see below).

Burn dressings
Practice varies from one hospital to another:

Exposure method:
- normally for face, buttocks, perineum
- antibacterial cream or iodine spray applied
- isolation if hospitalised.

Occlusive method:
- plastic bag or glove applied over hand covered in anti-bacterial cream. May require changing 3-4 times in first 48 hours when tissue fluid accumulates. *NB* Not used on small children who could smother themselves or bite through the bag.

- dressings:
  - transparent adhesive occlusive dressings which remain in place until the burn heals
  - simple paraffin gauze and dry dressings bandaged in place. Left in situ for up to a week if they remain dry and odourless
  - anti-bacterial burn cream (check for allergy to sulphonamides). Applied to wound with sterile spatula or gloved hand, or spread on non-adherent dressing which will cover the wound.

N.B. Rigorous adherence to aseptic technique is vital in dressing burns, preferably in a separate room or theatre area.

Transfer/discharge from A & E

Regional : For most burns over 30% area, or requiring urgent
Burns Centre plastic surgery.
Theatre : Burns of the *eyelids*, to prevent contracture
Head and neck burns, for tracheostomy
Small *electrical burns of the hand*, for immediate excision of the burn and skin-grafting
Circumferential burns of limbs, for incision of the "eschar" (constricting burn scar) which acts as a tourniquet
Burns of the *ears*, for excision and grafting of the burn to prevent deformity.
Ward : Most burns of over 5% in children or 10% in adults
Any burn in a child suspected of being non-accidental
Burns of both hands
Burns of the perineum
Extensive burns of the face or neck
Burns of the feet
Smoke inhalation.
Home : Small partial-thickness burns.

Advice to patient on discharge
- Elevate limb burns to reduce swelling
- Drink plenty of fluids
- Take adequate pain-killing tablets
- Do not get dressings wet or dirty
- Return to A & E (or GP) when instructed for dressings to be checked
- Take full course of antibiotics if prescribed.

The nurse has a role in educating patients and their relatives in prevention. Advice should be given regarding adequate preventive measures to ensure that the circumstances leading to the present injury are not repeated.

20 Less common injuries

Some injuries do not fit into any of the categories dealt with in the previous chapters. The aims of treatment of these injuries however are still the same:
- to prevent complications
- to restore function
- to relieve pain
- to ascertain cause and so help to prevent recurrence.

Crush injuries
These dangerous injuries result from a limb (usually) being trapped under pressure in a machine, in a vehicle following a crash, or under fallen masonry. The danger is due to:
- liberation of *myoglobin* from injured muscle, which causes kidney failure
- death of crushed tissue and *infection*
- hypovolaemic *shock*.

Assessment
- nature of injury (cause)
- length of time limb trapped (if for many hours amputation may be necessary)
- colour and condition of skin (clue to extent of tissue damage)
- pulse, blood pressure
- test urine for protein, blood, myoglobin
- measure urine output
- haemoglobin, urea and electrolytes.

Treatment
- elevation and ice-packs
- i-v fluids
- antibiotics and ATT
- analgesia
- operation to remove dead tissue.

Skin loss injuries
Caused by:
- lacerations (sharp instrument or broken glass)
- industrial accidents (e.g. hair caught in machinery)
- run over (by slow, heavy vehicle).

Skin may be lost entirely or partially, or sheared off from its deep attachments. If the skin is entirely torn off a finger (degloving), amputation may be required, or sometimes immediate skin-grafting. The main immediate problems are *blood loss* and *infection*. The patient needs:
- sterile dressings
- analgesia
- antibiotics
- ATT
- i-v fluids.

Bites
The mouths of people and animals are full of bacteria. These injuries (which include lacerations on the knuckles caused by punching someone in the mouth) are therefore likely to result in severe infection. Some animals (parrots, dogs, cats) can transmit specific infections through a bite. There is no rabies in Britain.

Treatment
- Elevation of affected part
- Antibiotics (first dose intramuscular, to obtain high blood level)
- ATT
- Plaster backslab to rest limb
- *Delayed suture* of wounds (patient returns after 4-5 days) to avoid infection
- Admission if injury severe, or late presentation with established infection.

Stab wounds
Damage depends on depth weapon has penetrated (sometimes estimated by size of wound and shape of knife). Normally patient is admitted for observation and may require exploration under GA. If the weapon is still in place, it is *not* removed in A & E: this might dislodge a clot plugging a blood vessel.

Self-inflicted lacerations
Usually multiple superficial cuts on front of left forearm (in right-handed person), or on side of neck. Previous similar healed wounds may be present. Patient may require admission, suture and psychiatric referral. Such patients are often reluctant to be treated and refuse admission and follow-up.

Electrical injuries
Depending on the current and site on injury, these may cause:
- burns (Chapter 19)
- heart arrythmias or cardiac arrest (Chapter 3)
- respiratory failure (Chapter 4)
- thrombosis of blood vessels
- shock.

Treatment:
- oxygen
- i-v fluids
- treatment of burn (usually full thickness).

Frostbite
Patients are usually vagrants or drug addicts "sleeping rough" in winter. They may also have hypothermia (see Chapter 5). Damaged capillaries result in thrombosis and gangrene.
Treatment
- slow re-warming
- i-v fluids
- antibiotics
- sometimes amputation.

"Superglue" injuries
This bonds firmly to skin; gentle soaking in warm soapy water allows the surfaces to be separated — do not try to pull them apart! A blunt instrument such as a spoon handle may be used in a sideways stroking action. Saliva softens the glue: if the lips are affected encourage the patient to salivate (e.g. by sucking on a sweet).

Tar and bitumen injuries
Adherent tar or bitumen requires Swarfega, oil of eucalyptus or liquid anaesthetic to aid removal. Burns may require appropriate local treatment (see Chapter 19).

Strangulation
Aim of treatment is to restore respiratory and circulatory function. After attempted strangling swelling of the neck tissues may endanger the airway.

Traumatic amputations
Of a whole limb: rare. Dangers are severe shock and infection; patient may be transferred to specialist centre
Of a finger or toe (whole or part): common (industrial or gardening accidents).

Assessment
- other injuries?
- is patient shocked?
- is replantation a possibility?

The last depends on:
- — part involved
- — level of injury
- — clean or contaminated wound
- — age and occupation
- — time since injury
- — facilities available (including experience of surgeon).

While a decision is being made it is important to maintain viability of the severed part, by placing it dry in a plastic bag surrounded by ice (to reduce the tissues' metabolic requirements).

Bleeding tooth socket

Patients usually attend some hours after a dental extraction.
    predisposing factors:
- — hypertension
- — anticoagulants
- — haemophilia
- — other bleeding disorders.

Treatment
- Spit out blood (irritant to stomach, causes vomiting)
- Rinse mouth
- Socket is packed with oxycel gauze (haemostatic)
- Bite hard for 10 minutes on gauze roll wrung out in hot water
- Socket is sutured with catgut (absorbable) under LA
- Refer patient to dentist following day.

For other dental problems, your Department will carry a list of dentists available for emergencies.

Broken teeth — may be reimplanted within an hour or so of damage. Pain relief: oil of cloves and zinc oxide paste. Oral surgeon may advise.

Dental abscess — analgesia, antibiotics, and referral to own dentist.

Nosebleeds (epistaxis)

Commoner in children and older people, and in those with bleeding tendencies (see above).

Treatment
- Reassurance
- Direct pressure by pinching nose for 10 minutes
- Suction to remove clots
- Pressure inside nostril with gauze pads soaked in vasoconstrictor solution (e.g. 10% cocaine)

- If bleeding from back of nose, insertion of 'posterior nasal pack'. A roll of gauze is tied to the end of a Foley catheter which has been passed through the nose into the pharynx. The gauze is then pulled back up through the mouth into the back of the nose.

Injuries to arteries and veins

Recognition of arterial injury
- Increasing pain and whiteness of a limb after fracture or laceration
- Absent pulse
- Rapidly enlarging swelling (which can cause dangerous pressure in the closed space of a limb).

Assessment
- Pulse and blood pressure
- Haemoglobin and cross-match
- Arteriogram (X-ray after injection of contrast medium).

Treatment
- Pressure bandaging over a sterile pad
- Elevation
- I-v fluids
- Transfer to theatre.

The commonest venous injury is rupture of a varicose vein, which stops with elevation and pressure. In elderly patients in particular, there may be significant blood loss if they have been unable to summon help quickly.

Paraphimosis

The foreskin is retracted and cannot be replaced, usually following intercourse. Treatment is by firm compression over an ice-pack, hyaluronidase injections or incision of the constricting tissue under GA.

Penetrating injuries and foreign bodies

Needle in the foot. Sometimes part of the needle has broken off. Requires X-ray (with paper-clip taped to the skin as a marker) and removal under GA in theatre.

Fish-hook in the skin. Removed by pushing onward in same direction (under LA) until the barb emerges. This is then cut off and the rest of the hook withdrawn.

Glass fragments. Frequently show on X-ray. Nerves and tendons may be damaged. Usually explored and removed under GA unless very superficial.

Wood splinters. Nearly always cause infection and require removal, ATT and antibiotics.

Airgun pellets. Require removal (usually under GA), especially if lying close to a blood vessel or nerve.

Transfixion injuries. (e.g. hand nailed to board, pitchfork passing through foot). These are rare, dramatic, and look deceptively easy to deal with. But sudden removal can cause severe haemorrhage, as the object may have been pressing on a blood vessel. Removal under GA is required.

Inhaled foreign bodies
- Small children — peanut or small toy
- Adults — fish- or chicken-bone.

Priority action
- Check **Airway**
- Reassure patient
- Throat examined by *laryngoscopy*
- *Bronchoscopy* under GA may be required.

Swallowed foreign bodies
- Small children — coins, beads, safety pins
- Mentally disturbed adults — various household items.

Most smooth objects, once in the stomach, will pass safely out per rectum in 2-3 days. A child who has swallowed a coin is X-rayed at intervals as an out-patient until the coin is passed. More irregular objects may require observation in hospital, and possible laparotomy for removal.

Other foreign bodies
Patients may present with objects lodged in the vagina, rectum or other body orifices. These may require GA for removal, and sometimes operation.

All these patients, when being initially assessed by the nurse, must be told not to eat or drink as this may delay treatment if an anaesthetic is required.

21 Injured children

Accidents are the largest single cause of death between the ages of 1 and 15. Children are usually injured:
— at home (e.g. limb fractures, head injury, scalds, cuts)
— at play (e.g. fractured forearm)
— on the road, where most of the fatal accidents occur (e.g. head, chest and abdominal injury, fractured femur or tibia).
Injured children recover better than adults: through further growth there is more potential to correct the damage.

Growing bones fracture differently from adult bones. They are pliable, not brittle; often only one side of a bone breaks ("greenstick fracture"). Damage to the ends of childrens' bones (the epiphyses) can lead to growth disturbances and are especially important.

Children are not small adults, and must not be treated as such. They have special needs in A & E (see also Chapter 11). They are frightened and disorientated by the strange surroundings, as well as by their injury. For the smaller child, detailed explanations of investigations and treatment are inappropriate, but a child should still be told what is happening next. This is very important. Gaining the child's confidence is vital; any sudden unannounced action (e.g. putting on a dressing) will lose it, probably for good. Demonstrate on a toy or on the parent so the child understands what is going to happen.

Do not separate the child from the parent who can help with reassurance, undressing and communication. Find out if your hospital allows a parent to stay overnight with a child; this is often the first thing a parent asks if a child is being admitted.

If he has not brought one, give the child a toy or cuddly animal to hold. If you have a separate play area take the child there. If possible, let him take a toy with him to theatre or the ward.

Ideally, the same nurse should stay with the child throughout. He will respond much better to one person with whom a relationship has been developed than to several different people. Try to find out the child's nickname, and use it or his first name frequently.

A badge or bravery certificate may help the child to remember hospital positively.

Get down to the child's level — a huge adult towering over a child is bound to be frightening!

If medicine has to be given, ask the parent whether a dropper, spoon or syringe is most acceptable. Firmness may be needed. The child may take the medicine more readily from the parent. Do not mix medicines with essential foods such as milk or cereal.

- If giving an injection, prepare and check it well away from the bedside
- Do not give an injection into the buttock as the muscle is not well developed; the thigh is the best site
- Tell the child what you are doing immediately before, hold him firmly, and administer the injection having warned him that it will hurt for a minute.

Take the opportunity of an A & E attendance to ensure a child is up to date with immunisations.

No child under 16 should be examined or treated in the absence of a parent or guardian, except in an emergency.

A GA is often required for even minor procedures in a child, where an adult could tolerate treatment under LA. It is therefore essential that all children are kept 'nil by mouth' until treatment is complete.

The great majority of injuries to children are accidental, *but some are not*. These are a vitally important minority; missing this diagnosis could have a fatal outcome.

Non-accidental injuries (NAI)
Physical violence against children occurs everywhere, and in all social classes. It is never easy to diagnose; nursing staff are often better at this than doctors. These are some features which should sound a warning:

- unlikely explanation for the injury ("bumped his head on the cot" to explain a skull fracture; "she bruises easily" to explain multiple soft-tissue injuries)
- apathetic, unkempt, under-nourished child, who shrinks from contact with adults
- severe nappy rash
- delay between injury and presentation at A & E
- evidence of previous injuries (bruises of different colours; other healing fractures on X-ray)
- apparent lack of parental concern; alternatively over-defensive attitude
- history of frequent A & E attendances
- specific injuries:
    scalds of buttocks, thighs, feet
    cigarette burns
    multiple bruises (especially head and neck)
    finger imprint bruises
    rib fractures

injury to the mucosa of the upper lip
evidence of sexual abuse (e.g. genital bruising and lacerations).
Most A & E departments keep a confidential register of children
"at risk" . . . . . but there is always a first time, and there are those
who have slipped through the net.

If NAI is suspected the child is gently and carefully fully
undressed and examined. X-rays of the chest, skull and all four
limbs may be requested, to look for evidence of previous injuries.

Any suggestion that an injury might be non-accidental will
provoke great resentment in the parent: tact and understanding are
vital. As the diagnosis of NAI is so serious (for both child and
parent), genuine accidental causes of repeated injury *must* be
carefully excluded (e.g. bleeding disorders, fragile bone disease). If
NAI is strongly suspected, every effort is made to admit the child,
regardless of the type of injury. Urgent referrals are made to the
paediatrician, social worker, GP and community health team, and
sometimes the police.

The present and future safety of the child is the over-riding
concern in this distressing situation.

The attendance of a child at A & E presents an excellent
opportunity for advising the parents on relevant accident prevention
measures, e.g.:
fire guards
cooker guards
stair gates
window locks
cupboard locks
matches and medicines out of reach
cycling proficiency training
car child restraints.

22 Wound management, bandaging, plaster and appliances

WOUND MANAGEMENT

Of primary importance in handling patients with open wounds is protection of the nurse against infection, especially:
• Hepatitis
• AIDS.
Measures required:
• gloves
• plastic apron
• proper disposal of linen, rubbish, sharps
• thorough cleansing of surfaces and equipment between patients
• package laboratory specimens carefully:
  — check tops/lids
  — place in plastic bag
  — if high risk, attach label to warn laboratory.

Wound care
Initially all wounds require thorough cleansing with cetrimide solution and/or peroxide.

Suitable wound management
• Exposure only — small cuts and grazes
• Dry iodine spray — more extensive grazes, small skin breaks
• Non-adherent dry dressings
• Skin closure strips — small superficial lacerations, especially on delicate skin
• Paraffin gauze (with or without antibacterial agent), and dry dressings
• Occlusive adhesive air-permeable plastic film
• Suturing: this is an extended role undertaken only by a trained A & E nurse or a doctor. Local or regional anaesthesia is required (see Appendix A). Plastic spray or a dry dressing is usually applied
• Tetanus prophylaxis:
  — booster dose of anti-tetanus toxoid (ATT) if no dose in past 5 years

   — commence full course (ATT stat and at 6 weeks and 6
     months) if no dose in past 10 years
   — human tetanus immunoglobulin for patients with highly
     contaminated wounds and no prior protection
 • Antibiotics — intramuscular or oral may be prescribed.
The simplest and least bulky dressing is best as the patient usually
has to return home or to work. The bulkier the dressing the less
likely the patient is to keep it on.

Attachment of dressings
 • Adhesive strip dressings — easy for patient to renew
 • Conforming adhesive tape which holds well on awkward
   surfaces, e.g. axilla, heels
 • Cotton/rayon conforming bandage — cheap, comfortable, cool
 • Cotton tubular bandage for fingers and toes
 • Crepe bandage — expensive and unnecessary except where
   pressure or compression required.

Advice to patient on discharge
 • Elevate affected part
 • Take full course of antibiotics as prescribed
 • Leave dressings in place
 • Keep dressings/wound clean and dry
 • Take simple pain relief (e.g. paracetamol) as required
 • Complete tetanus vaccination course if previously unprotected
 • Return to A & E or attend GP if wound becomes inflamed or
   more painful, or discharges
 • Keep follow-up appointment for change of dressing or removal of
   sutures.

BANDAGING

Used to support most sprains, strains and soft-tissue injuries not
severe enough to require immobilisation in plaster, and also some
minor fractures. Most of these injuries will be expected to heal in
2-3 weeks. The bandaging may need to be re-applied several times,
by a community or practice nurse, relative or the patient himself.

> **Make sure the patient is not allergic to adhesive bandages before
> applying.**

The following rules apply when bandaging:
 • not too tight
 • "position of safe splintage" (see Figure 2) for bandaging the
   hand
 • elbow and ankle at 90 degrees.

   Ankle strapping (sprained ankle). Adhesive strapping over tubular
cotton bandage. Applied round foot, ankle and lower leg (to top of

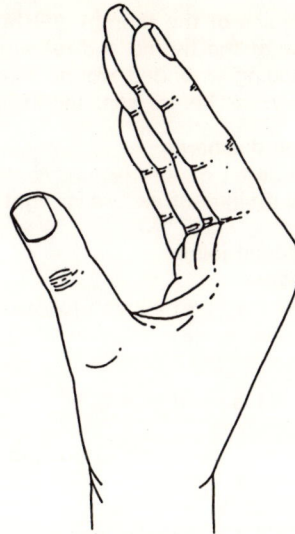

Fig. 2   The "position of safe splintage". (Reproduced from Watson N 1985 Practical management of musculoskeletal emergencies. Oxford: Blackwell Scientific Publications, by permission of the author and publisher.)

the calf) in the direction which will tend to turn the foot outwards (sprains are usually caused by twisting the foot inwards).

Tubular elastic bandages are applied for minor strains and sprains. It is important to use the measuring tape supplied to ensure the correct size is fitted for maximum effect and safety. A double layer may be used for extra support.

Robert Jones bandage (knee ligament and cartilage injuries). Two or three layers of wool and crepe to provide pressure and support.

Tubular finger bandages are used to hold dressings in place and provide protective padding. Apply with cylindrical metal applicator ensuring correct size selected. Finish with tape to secure, or split and tie ends finishing around wrist or base of finger — *not too tight!*

"Boxing-glove bandage" (for e.g. fractured metacarpal). Crepe bandage over orthopaedic wool, with a roll of wool in the palm and padding between the fingers. Hand in "position of safe splintage" (see Figure 2).

Bedford splint (for e.g. reduced finger-joint dislocation, or finger fractures). "Siamesed" double tubular cotton bandage: uses an uninjured finger to support its injured neighbour. Alternative is neighbour strapping: padding inserted between fingers (or toes) and strapping to adjacent finger applied between joints.

Thumb spica (sprains of the thumb). "Fishtail" adhesive strapping to support the base of the thumb and restrict movement, with figure-of-eight strapping extended around thumb and wrist. Protect skin with tinct. benz. co. before applying strapping.

Advice to patient on discharge
• Elevate affected part
• Return to A & E if signs of excessive tightness develop (due to swelling)
• Exercise unbandaged joints
• Keep bandages dry
• Tubular bandages may be removed for washing.

PLASTER

Plaster of Paris (p.o.p.) is used in A & E:
• as emergency splintage
• to hold fractures and dislocations reduced
• to support soft-tissue injuries
• to protect a repaired nerve or tendon
• to prevent movement in an inflamed or infected part.
Other types of "synthetic casting material" are sometimes used. Because it sets hard *plaster can be dangerous:*
• causing pressure sores on bony prominences
• constricting a swollen limb, cutting off the blood supply.
   The technique of applying plaster is an extended nursing role requiring careful training. This chapter only draws attention to the most important points. Once these are understood, relevant advice (see below) can be given to the patient.
   The patient's confidence and cooperation are essential. Ensure he is sitting (or lying) comfortably. Remove rings or jewellery, and *all* clothing on the affected limb. Clean any lacerations or abrasions and dress with simple non-adherent dressings and minimal taping.
   You may be asked to support the patient's limb while the plaster is being applied.
— do not use finger-tips: they may indent wet plaster
— support the plaster with the flat of the hand.

Note
• it is important to pad the skin well (with no wrinkles) especially over prominent bones (wrist, ankle)
• a complete plaster is usually "split" lengthways when set — with a knife or electric saw — to allow for swelling
• plaster must be washed off patient's skin and clothing after cast has been applied
• a "check X-ray" may be taken to ensure the procedure has not altered the position of a fracture
• the patient is given advice on care of the limb in plaster (see below).

A limb (or part of a limb) can be protected in a plaster "backslab", which is less likely to cause dangerous constriction, but is not as strong as a complete plaster.

Advice to patient with a plaster cast

This is perhaps the most important part of the whole procedure. The patient (or parent) must be clearly told to:

- Return immediately if the fingers (or toes) become blue, numb, or increasingly swollen or painful
- Avoid getting the plaster wet (advise the patient to cover the plaster with a plastic bag when washing)
- Avoid walking on a "walking plaster" for 48 hours; although it feels hard in half-an-hour or less it takes much longer to develop its full strength
- Elevate the limb to reduce swelling (arm in a sling, leg so that the foot is higher than the hip. The leg must be evenly supported so the plaster does not get indented)
- Expose to air to aid drying; do not apply heat (e.g. hair-dryer) or sit near fire
- Never put anything down inside the plaster (it could cause a pressure sore)
- Return if the plaster cracks, breaks or softens
- *Exercise all unsplinted joints regularly,* e.g. shoulder and elbow in forearm plaster; ankle and foot in plaster cylinder
- *Exercise all muscles regularly inside plaster,* e.g. thigh muscles by lifting up leg, then lowering it slowly
- Return for A & E or clinic appointment as requested
- Take simple pain relief (e.g. paracetamol) as required.

APPLIANCES

Sling. Cotton triangle folded and tied to one side of the neck, to support an injured forearm horizontally ("broad-arm sling") or with the hand elevated ("high-arm sling"). The sling must support the hand to the finger-tips.

Collar-and-cuff. Lengths of cotton-covered sponge looped over the neck and wrist and clipped together. This leaves the elbow free and allows the weight of the arm to produce traction.

Crutches. The right length is 5 cm (2 in) less than the height of the patient's axilla from the ground. The patient must be taught to take his weight on his hands, not axillae, and swing forwards not more than 30 cm (12 in) at a time. He must be seen to be safe on crutches, and the condition of the screws and rubber ferrules must be checked, before discharge from A & E.

Walking stick. The right length is the height of the patient's wrist from the ground with the arm by the side. The stick is held on the uninjured side (except on stairs). Instruction on the use of a stick is given, and the condition of the rubber ferrule is checked, before discharge from A & E.

Collar. A. "soft collar" (padded sponge) or "hard collar" (moulded plastic) may be prescribed for neck injuries, e.g. whiplash. The collar should be worn all the time (except for washing) or as directed by the doctor. Select a collar that fits firmly but not too tightly and is in no danger of causing local pressure (back of skull, angles of jaw). Keep collar clean by covering with length of stockinette.

Corset. Plaster rooms carry supplies of "instant" corsets in standard sizes, for patients with minor back injuries not requiring admission. Patients with a history of indigestion or acid regurgitation may be unable to tolerate a corset. The corset should be worn all the time during the day, or as directed by the doctor.

Skin traction. This may be set up in A & E, prior to the patient's transfer to the ward, usually for a fractured neck of femur (Chapter

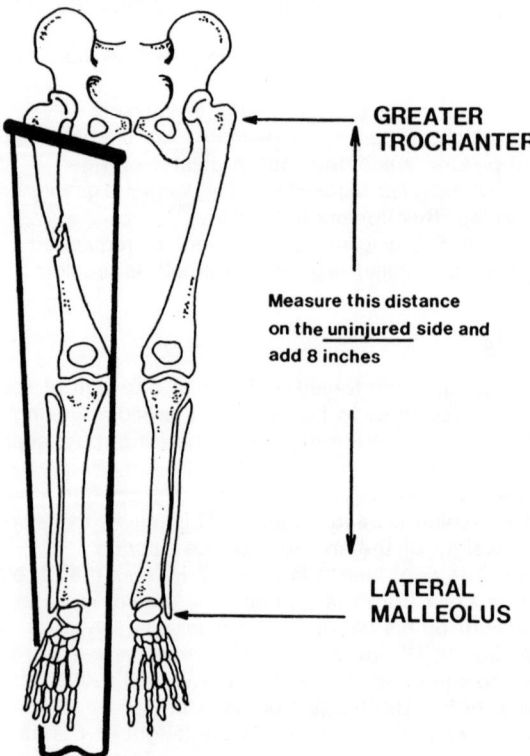

GREATER TROCHANTER

Measure this distance on the <u>uninjured</u> side and add 8 inches

LATERAL MALLEOLUS

Fig. 3   Taking the measurements for a Thomas splint.

17) or low back pain (Chapter 18). Non-adhesive traction sets with foam-backed fabric are used which protect the skin. A crepe or cotton bandage holds the traction in position. Weights (2.3 kg (5 lb) maximum) can be attached directly to the traction cord which is fixed to the base of the spreader under the foot.

Thomas splint. This is a metal frame used (with appropriate slings) to support an injured lower limb, usually a fractured shaft of femur (see Figure 3).

Measurements (on the uninjured side) required to select a Thomas splint are:
— thigh circumference: add 3-4 inches to allow for swelling unless splint ring adjustable
— limb length: greater trochanter to lateral malleolus plus 8 inches
— note if left or right-sided splint required: ensure you get the right one for the injured limb.

The preparation and application of a Thomas splint can only be learned by practical experience. Larger books describe the procedure fully.

Appendix A

Pain relief in A & E

Recognition of pain is vital — it is apparent in an obviously injured patient, but may not be recognised in the baby or young child, the mentally handicapped, or those with speech or language difficulty.

Signs of pain include:
— restlessness
— crying/whimpering
— unwillingness to allow examination.

Pain is part of almost every patient's reason for attendance at A & E. A patient whose pain is relieved is less frightened, more confident, and more able to cooperate in their nursing care. While pain relief (analgesia) is an important function of A & E treatment, its nature and location are often vital clues to diagnosis.

Factors affecting pain
- fear
- culture
- previous experience
- in children, the parents' attitude has a significant effect.

The many ways of preventing or reducing pain in the ill or injured patient can be summarised as:

(a) Physical
- careful and gentle removal of clothing
- support/splintage of a fracture (e.g. backslab, Thomas splint)
- limitation of movement — use radiotranslucent stretcher/mattress to avoid the need to move patient for X-ray
- elevation to reduce swelling and therefore pain
- application of ice, e.g. to swollen ankle
- application of cold wet sterile pads to burns.

(b) Psychological
A calm, informed patient will be better able to cope with pain and may be less affected by it.
- information — what is likely to happen and length of wait (especially for minor injuries). A translator or language cards may be useful

- distraction — listen to the patient, respond and stay with him
- physical contact — cuddle a baby; hold a confused elderly patient's hand.

(c)   Drugs
- analgesia (inhalational, oral, intramuscular, intravenous or rectal)
- local anaesthesia (LA)
- regional anaesthesia
- general anaesthesia (GA).

Anaesthesia means "lack of feeling"; *analgesia* specifically means "lack of pain".
N.B.Many patients do not understand the term 'analgesia'.

Analgesia

In some circumstances analgesia can be positively dangerous. In *head injuries* (Chapter 14) narcotic drugs — e.g. pethidine, morphine, omnopon — depress consciousness and obscure the patient's true condition. Narcotics also depress respiration, and in *chest injuries* (Chapter 15) or *acute respiratory problems* (Chapter 4) they make the patient iller with a greater chance of developing pneumonia.

Inhalational
Entonox, a *self-administered* 50/50 mixture of nitrous oxide and oxygen, is widely used in A & E and by ambulance crews. It is effective and safe (the patient himself must hold the mask to his face: as he begins to lose consciousness the mask will fall away and he no longer breathes the gas). Also, the high oxygen content is beneficial in the severely injured patient.

Oral
Tablets or liquid (for children). Simple, slow-acting (e.g. aspirin, paracetamol, co-proxamol etc.). Usually prescribed for minor injuries, to take home. Aspirin is not given to children under 12 (risk of Reye's Syndrome). Explain dosage to patient before discharge.

Intramuscular
Narcotic (see above) or non-narcotic drugs. The commonest route of analgesic administration in A & E. Acts in 15-30 minutes, lasts up to 4-6 hours.

Intravenous
For severe pain (myocardial infarction, burns). A steady, continuous level of pain relief is achieved. No delay in effect, and better in a shocked patient who absorbs an intramuscular drug poorly because of low blood flow to muscles.

Rectal
Suitable for children, e.g. pre-medication.

Local anaesthesia
Commonly used for minor procedures e.g. suturing of lacerations.
Lignocaine used for subcutaneous injection comes in:
— 0.5%, 1% or 2% strengths
— *with or without adrenaline.*
Adrenaline constricts small arteries, so prevents dissipation of the
drug, but *can cause gangrene* if accidentally injected *into* an artery.
It is therefore never used on fingers or toes. Lignocaine takes 5
minutes to act and lasts about 30-60 minutes.

Surface (topical) anaesthesia (ether-based spray which "freezes"
the skin). Occasionally used for very localised, very short-acting
pain relief, e.g. splinter removal.

Infiltration of fracture haematoma with lignocaine; occasionally
used for reduction of e.g. metacarpal or Colles fractures.

Regional anaesthesia
Pain relief over a wide area by "blocking" the nerves supplying the
part, with LA solution.

Examples:
- "Ring block" — LA injections (*no adrenaline*) around the nerves
  at the base of a finger or toe anaesthetise the whole digit.
- "Brachial block" — LA injections around the brachial plexus
  (nerves of the upper limb) in the neck or axilla anaesthetise the
  whole limb.
- "Intercostal block" — LA injection around the intercostal nerves
  provide analgesia in rib fractures. This improves breathing, and
  permits physiotherapy.
- "Bier's block" — LA injection into forearm veins after blood has
  been drained from limb and an upper arm tourniquet applied.
  Used for minor hand operations and reduction of Colles
  fractures.

General anaesthesia
Depending on your Department's facilities, GA may be given in
A & E; otherwise the patient is transferred to theatre. GA is
required for most open operations, and for some fracture
reductions, especially in children.

Important points:
- When did the patient last eat or drink (even a cup of tea)?
  Except in dire emergency GA is withheld for 4-6 hours after the
  last oral intake. This ensures the stomach has emptied and there
  is less danger of vomiting and inhalation. Gastric absorption
  often ceases after an accident

- Ensure patient remains strictly "nil by mouth" in A & E
- Check regular medications and allergies
- Record pulse and blood pressure
- Remove rings and jewellery — store according to valuables procedure
- Undress patient and put on theatre gown
- Bag and label all patient's possessions
- Put on identity bracelet
- Weigh patient if possible, or ask his weight (often unreliable)
- Test urine
- ECG and chest X-ray in the elderly
- Sickle-cell test for negro patients
- Remove false teeth; check and note crowns
- Check consent form signed.

After a GA a patient is either admitted, or discharged several hours later, *accompanied by a responsible adult.*

Advice to patient on discharge after GA
- Do not drive or operate machinery for 24 hours
- Do not take alcohol for 24 hours
- Avoid smoking (danger of pneumonia)
- Return if vomiting or severe headaches occur. (See also Chapter 22: Advice to patient in plaster).

Appendix B

Social and legal problems

Anne James BA MA IMSW
Social Worker, Nuffield Orthopaedic Centre, Oxford
Formerly Social Worker, Accident Service, John Radcliffe Hospital, Oxford

A busy A & E department can seem threatening to an ill or injured patient and his relatives. Admission to A & E is just one incident in your patient's total life. Many people presenting with illness and injury already have immense and complicated personal and social problems which are compounded by the emotional and physical implications of their immediate condition. The patient's psychological and social responses to A & E attendance are as important as the clinical features.

* patients will tell you a lot of personal details they would normally never admit to
* they will seek reassurances — that you cannot give — about what is wrong and what will happen to them
* they may be aggressive, angry, and even violent, especially if they are kept waiting.

How do you cope?
* **Never** offer false reassurances, or a diagnosis
* **Think** about which social and personal problems can be sorted out "on the spot" (probably very few, if any)
* **Listen** to verbal anger and aggression without defending yourself or your hospital
* **Offer comfort and support** in a "non-directive" way; by holding the patient's hand, giving him a hug, or just staying and listening
* **Tell** the nurse in charge any social or personal problems the patient has told you about.

Confidentiality is vital

When considering *discharge* or *transfer* from A & E find out:
* where is the patient going to?
* who will look after him in the short term (tonight, tomorrow, over the weekend), and in the longer term? Do those who are going to look after him understand the implications of the injury or illness?

- how is the injury or illness going to affect the patient's day-to-day life?
- will he or she be mentally and physically safe? Is there a risk of further injury, either self-inflicted or inflicted by others, e.g. a violent husband?

Sometimes a social worker, health visitor or the GP can help with these problems; sometimes admission is advisable (other than for medical reasons).

Confusion and disorientation

In addition to medical causes and head injuries this state may be due to the unfamiliar surroundings of A & E (especially in the elderly).

Old people

Most live alone, or with another elderly person. The questions above about discharge are particularly relevant here. For instance, your patient with a Colles' fracture won't be able to open a tin, help a wheelchair-bound husband, or use a walking aid.

Ethnic minorities

People whose first language is not English will often have difficulty understanding what is happening to them in hospital, however thorough the explanation. A culturally acceptable translator (preferably of the same sex) is essential in caring for these patients in A & E. Often an accompanying friend or relative can do this.

Hospitals in areas with large immigrant populations may have staff who can act as translators. Local Community Relations Councils or ethnic minority welfare groups can also supply interpreters. Language- or picture-cards, if available, may also be helpful.

Sensitivity to the customs of other cultures is important. Muslim women, for example, are not supposed to be seen by any man other than their husband, and it may be upsetting for them to be required to undress for examination.

Road traffic accidents

You can help by:

- finding out who needs contacting (relative, friend)
- reassuring the patient that the police will deal with the vehicle and its contents
- informing the nurse in charge if relatives and friends wish to stay overnight. The Department may have a list of readily available accommodation nearby. Sometimes a bed may be available in the hospital for the relative of a seriously ill or injured patient.

Child abuse (see also Chapter 21)

If there is any suspicion that a child may have been physically or

sexually abused, he or she should be admitted at least overnight.
Parents do not usually refuse to allow a child to be admitted. If they
do it may be necessary to obtain a *Place of Safety Order.* The
childrens' wards of most hospitals are designated as "places of
safety", and once a child is the subject of an Order it is an offence
to remove him from the place of safety. To obtain a Place of Safety
Order, which needs to be signed by a magistrate, one of the
following has to be contacted:
— hospital social worker, during office hours
— duty social worker, outside office hours
— the police; some areas have nominated senior policewomen to
   act as liaison officers in such cases.

Rape
Women who have been raped, or feel they have been raped even if
there is no conclusive evidence, may be very withdrawn, or they
may be severely agitated. Rape affects different women in different
ways. It is important to accept the woman's story, even if it does
not seem wholly credible, and to reassure her that the rape was not
her fault. Many women suffer years of guilt, believing that they
provoked the rape.

Often women do not want to report a rape, and they should be
given that option. If a woman *does* wish to report a rape, she will
need to undergo an internal examination by a police doctor in order
to provide forensic evidence.

All rape victims should be advised to contact their GP for sexually
transmitted disease screening and pregnancy testing. They can insist
on seeing a woman GP for this even if there is not one in their practice.

Many areas have a Rape Crisis phone line which offers support
and counselling to victims.

Services providing social help
Hospital social workers specialise in the social implications of illness
and injury and can offer counselling, support, and financial and
material help and guidance. A "samaritan fund" is usually available
for small immediate cash problems, e.g. taxi fares. Through the
Social Security Office, emergency cash payments or payment for
bed-and-breakfast or hostel accommodation can also be arranged.
Outside normal working hours there is emergency cover by a
community-based duty social worker.

If a patient dies in A & E
In this difficult situation the news must be broken gently by a
senior member of staff to the next-of-kin or those accompanying
the patient. If there is any doubt regarding identification it may be
necessary to ask one of the relatives to identify the deceased in the
presence of a police officer. Any relatives or friends with the
patient will need comfort and support.

The initial stage of the grief reaction is often numbness and disbelief. Viewing the body may be requested and may help relatives to come to terms with the situation. The religion of the deceased should be established in case special observances are required. The relatives may wish contact to be made with a minister of their religion. Practical measures such as providing a cup of tea and paper tissues are appreciated.

If young children are present, as in the case of a cot death, you may be asked to look after them for a while.

Sudden death is always reported to the coroner, so it is important that the relatives are warned that the police will be contacting them. They will also need practical help with the process of registering the death, claiming the death grant and making funeral arrangements. The subject of organ donation may arise and is dealt with by senior staff.

Consents for treatment

Most adults can consent for their own treatment (e.g. operation). Some people however cannot, and it is important to know how to go about obtaining consents for them.

Children under 16 need the consent of a parent or guardian for treatment (e.g. operation). If a child under 16 is in the care of the Local Authority Social Service Department, the parents will usually have signed a form on his reception into care allowing his social worker or Head of Home (if he is in a Childrens' Home or Community Home) to sign a consent form to authorise treatment.

These procedures also apply to children living with foster parents (but not adopted children), and Wards of Court.

Children at a boarding school usually come with a School Nurse or Matron, who is often authorised to sign a consent form.

Refusal of consent by parents. In these special circumstances the doctor in charge of the child's treatment may proceed without parental consent (e.g. in life-saving situations) provided he obtains the written support of a medical colleague, and establishes that the parent or guardian will not consent to treatment.

Adults held under certain Sections of the Mental Health Act may be deemed by that Act to be not responsible for their actions and therefore unable to consent to their own treatment. This is commonly called *"being under Section"*. A doctor or a senior nurse will need to obtain consent on the patient's behalf. A psychiatrist, social worker, or the patient's next-of-kin can in this instance consent on the patient's behalf.

Conclusion

The less time anyone spends in hospital the better. Try to build up a picture of the patient's total life prior to admission, and match it to the current situation. The hospital and community caring services can then ensure he is discharged as quickly as possible into the optimal physical and social environment.

Glossary

You may already know many of these terms. You will certainly meet them whilst working in the Accident and Emergency Department, and it is important to understand them.

Abduction   Movement away from the mid-line of the body.

Adduction   Movement towards the mid-line of the body.

Anaphylaxis   Severe sensitivity reaction to foreign protein (e.g. bee-sting, certain foods and drugs, especially antibiotics). May include dyspnoea, hypotension, loss of consciousness.

Bursitis   Inflammation in a burse (a sac of fluid lying between a tendon and a bone).

Callus   New bone formed in fracture healing.

Colles' fracture   Fracture of lower end of radius.

Comminuted   Bone broken into more than two pieces.

Compound   Fracture in communication with the outside through a wound.

Condyle   The end of a long bone forming part of a joint.

Crepitus   Grating of ends of fractured bones.

Debridement   Removal of devitalised tissue and foreign material from a wound.

Distal   Towards the periphery of the body.

Effusion   An excess of fluid in the tissues or in a body cavity.

Epicondyle   Protruding part of a long bone adjacent to a joint, where muscles are attached.

Epiphysis   The growing end of a bone before maturity.

Epistaxis   Nose-bleed.

Foetor   Unpleasant smell of breath in dehydrated patient with acute abdominal condition, e.g. appendicitis.

Haemarthrosis   Collection of blood in a joint.

Haematoma   Localised collection of blood in the tissues.

Hemiplegia   Paralysis of one side of the body; a form of stroke.

Internal fixation   Fracture fixation with screws, nails and plates at open operation.

Irritable hip   Painful hip in a child without definite diagnosis.

Kyphosis   Forward bending of the spine.

Lateral   Positioned away from the mid-line of the body.

Lordosis   Backward bending of the spine.

Malleoli   Bony prominences of the lower tibia and fibula forming the sides of the ankle joint.

Mallet finger   Injury to the extensor tendon at the terminal finger-joint causing the tip of the finger to drop.

Medial   Positioned towards the mid-line of the body.

Melaena   Black tarry stools due to the presence of altered blood.

Munchausen's syndrome   Repeated feigned illnesses resulting in hospital admissions and often operations.

Narcotics   Drugs producing profound sleep and pain relief; most are addictive, e.g. heroin.

Oblique   description of the line of a fracture in relation to the long axis of a bone.

Olecranon   Upper end of the ulna, forming part of the elbow joint.

Open reduction   Operation to replace fracture fragments in correct position.

Osteomyelitis   Infection of bone.

Palpitations   Awareness of the action of the heart.

Papilloedema   Oedema of the optic nerve seen through the ophthalmoscope; a sign of raised intracranial pressure.

Paraphimosis   Swelling of the penis due to a tight foreskin which has been retracted and cannot be replaced.

Paraplegia   Paralysis of the lower half of the body due to spinal injury or disease in the thoracic or lumbar region.

Paronychia   Infection of the edge of the nail-bed with abscess formation.

Pathological fracture   Fracture occurring in bone already weakened by disease, e.g. tumour.

Plantar   Towards the sole of the foot.

Plantar response   Reflex indicating integrity of the nerve tracts passing to the brain; stroking the sole of the foot normally causes the big toe to flex downwards.

Pott's fracture   Fracture-dislocation of the ankle.

Prone   Lying on the front.

Proximal   Towards the centre of the body.

Quadruplegia   Paralysis of all four limbs due to spinal injury or disease in the cervical region. Tetraplegia is the same.

Septic arthritis   Presence of pus in a joint.

Sciatica   Pain referred down the back of the leg from nerve root irritation in the back, e.g. by a prolapsed disc.

Scoliosis   Sideways curvature of the spine.

Shock   Inadequate tissue perfusion due to reduction in effective circulatory volume.

Spiral   Description of the line of a fracture in relation to the long axis of a bone.

Strangulation   Interference with the blood supply, usually of a hernia.

Stridor   Whistling sound on inspiration due to airway obstruction, e.g. in croup.

Subluxation   Partial dislocation of a joint.

Subungual   Beneath a nail.

Supine   Lying on the back.

Syncope   Fainting.

Tamponade   Constriction of the heart due to effusion in the pericardium.

Tetraplegia   See quadruplegia.

Transverse   Description of the line of a fracture in relation to the long axis of a bone.

Trephine (as in finger nail)   Make a hole through the nail with a blunt instrument to release a subungual haematoma.

Triage   Sorting of injured patients by degree of severity and urgency of treatment required.

Trocar   Sharp instrument used to assist the insertion of a tube through the skin.

Trochanter   Bony prominence on the upper femur.

Urticaria   Itchy allergic rash, often due to nettle or insect stings.
Vaso-vagal   Acute hypotensive attack resulting in loss of consciousness: the common "faint".
Volar   On the palmar surface of the hand or forearm.

Bibliography

It is obviously not possible to cover all aspects of Accident and Emergency nursing in detail in this small book. A number of other excellent texts are available; many have good illustrations. You may find the following helpful.

Bache J B, Armitt Carolyn R, Tobiss J Ruth 1985 A colour atlas of nursing procedures in accidents and emergencies. Wolfe Medical Publications, London.

Bradley D 1984 Accident and emergency nursing, 2nd edn. Balliere Tindall, London.

Huckstep R L 1978 A simple guide to trauma, 2nd edn. Churchill Livingstone, Edinburgh.

McRae R 1981 Practical fracture treatment. Churchill Livingstone, Edinburgh.

Mid-Glamorgan Health Authority, Wales 1984 Accident and emergency department guidelines and information document. King's Fund Centre, London.

Miller Margaret, Miller J H 1985 Orthopaedics and accidents illustrated. Hodder and Stoughton, London.

Mills K, Morton R, Page G 1984 A colour atlas of accidents and emergencies. Wolfe Medical Publications, London.

Walsh M 1985 Accident and emergency nursing. A new approach. Heinemann, London.

There is a good chapter on the Emergency Treatment of Poisoning in the British National Formulary.

Index